SUNBREAK

HEALING THE PAIN
NO ONE CAN EXPLAIN

By Shana Johnson, MD

Book design by Sarah Haynes, shareddrive.com

Cover art by Debra Van Tuinen, vantuinenart.com

Printed in the United States of America

First Edition

ISBN 9798860666337

While all the patient stories described in this book are based on true experiences, names and personal details have been changed to protect their privacy.

The information included in this book is for educational purposes only. It is not intended or implied to be a substitute for professional medical advice. The reader should always consult with a qualified healthcare provider to determine the appropriateness of the information for their own situation or for information regarding a medical condition or treatment plan. Reading the information in this book does not constitute a physician-patient relationship. The statements in this book are not intended to diagnose, treat, cure, or prevent any disease. The author expressly disclaims responsibility for any adverse effects that may result from the use or application of the information contained in this book.

For the readers, seeking
understanding and answers.

CONTENTS

CHAPTER 1

When the sun breaks through

WHEN I LIVED IN SEATTLE, the sky was gray for nine long months, from October through June. During this gloom, short bursts of sun appeared, lasting only a few hours. We called them "sunbreaks"—so rare they were considered events. These exciting moments delivered an invigorating break from the gray and gloom, as the sun reflected off the ocean and lit up the mountain ranges. No place is more beautiful than Seattle when the sun breaks free.

I remember the welcome sight of a sunbreak during the years I worked as a physical medicine and rehabilitation physician in the Seattle area. I focused mostly in the neurology world, treating people with conditions affecting the brain, spine, and nerves. Multiple sclerosis was a particular specialty of mine. I also cared for patients who had suffered severe brain injuries, spinal cord injuries, and strokes. And pain of all different types—back pain, headaches, and whole-body pain. I treated the vast spectrum of injury and recovery.

Throughout the years, I frequently encountered a condition that my medical training hadn't prepared me for: people who developed medical disorders while under long-standing overwhelming stress.

And, then, I developed one too.

My stress-related disorder (SRD) turned my life upside down. While devastating at the time, I can now feel the pain of 30 million Americans suffering from similar disorders.

The sun breaking free reminds me of finding hope and starting on a path toward healing. Finding light in the gloom. Realizing that dark days are temporary. These momentary flashes of sunlight inspired me to write this book on a subject close to my heart. *Sunbreak* offers insight and guidance for healing from medical conditions that are triggered and worsened by stress. Conditions like chronic headaches, back pain, bladder pain, and digestive issues, as well as depression and anxiety disorders triggered by trauma and overwhelming stress. As a doctor, I've seen too many patients with real and serious pain who were ignored, dismissed or misdiagnosed. I've also been one of those patients.

Follow me down the path from pain to wellness for several individuals—each on a different life path—who developed different medical conditions while under high stress. Each person faced significant losses because of their medical issues. Despite their individual life paths and conditions, their journeys to healing all contained the same key elements. And I want to share them with you so that you understand that there is hope for healing and you know where to find it.

I titled the book *Sunbreak* because this "enlightening" represents the first element of healing; the illumination that comes with awareness. Becoming aware of your mind, body, and self. And, more importantly, becoming aware of how they are connected.

At the time I developed my stress-related disorder, I was working as a physician at a multiple sclerosis center. The position had been my career goal, my dream job, and my definition of success. The future looked bright then. But it did not go as I had dreamed.

I started on my path toward healing there, in the Pacific Northwest, where my greatest success met my greatest failure.

CHAPTER 2

My story: I feel your pain

WORKING AS A PHYSICIAN AT the multiple sclerosis center was my career goal. Being promoted to co-director of the clinic was my dream job. My new title afforded a leadership position to improve the quality of the care patients received. To grow an environment where patients are heard and supported.

A month after my promotion, I received exciting news that I was pregnant with my first child. There were a few logistical issues to be sorted through. Added work demands and the two hour commute from the clinic were more complicated with a baby on the way. Nonetheless, I saw no problem making it work. I deeply wanted both the roles of motherhood and clinic co-director. I was determined to continue at a pace of one hundred percent commitment to my career and one hundred percent present for my child.

Yes, the numbers didn't add up. Math was not my strongest subject in school.

So, I turned to my lifelong love of books, learning, and self-improvement tapes. My husband urged me to listen to a Tony Robbins motivational tape. While driving to work, I played the tape. He enthusiastically spoke about being strong. He declared something like, "You can do it because you have to."

I connected to that phrase. I told myself, I will be able to balance my new job and a baby because I have to and I want to. Tony's phrase, coupled with my impressive denial of reality, convinced me my situation was doable. The distance, the intense job, the baby, no family support…no problem.

And the reality struck me with full force.

My son, Asher, was born a month premature. The delivery nurse remarked, "What a spunky little preemie," as she handed him to me. Asher was ready to join the world. Well, except for his lungs; his lungs were not ready.

After a three-month maternity leave, I intently returned to work. I had found a great daycare close to my clinic. Full of confidence, I dropped him off at daycare and told myself, "I got this", as I headed to work. I was oblivious to the risks of putting a premature newborn in daycare during respiratory syncytial virus (RSV) and flu season. Couldn't that have been mentioned in one of the eight or so newborn visits with my pediatrician over the last few months?

Cashing the first reality check

That Friday, I picked up Asher from daycare and felt him burning up in my arms. As I looked closer, I saw that he was having trouble breathing. Five days after returning to work, my premature newborn son was admitted to the hospital in respiratory distress caused by RSV. I spent the next week back at work in Seattle Children's Hospital. I had barely made it through one week in the clinic before I was gone again, in the hospital with Asher. It would take three to four months for his lungs to fully recover. The universe was trying to tell me my plans were not going to work, but I was still deep in denial. I didn't listen.

After the hospitalization, my pediatrician warned me that, as a result of the RSV infection, Asher would be at a higher risk of developing lung problems and specifically asthma. She was right. I don't think he ever stopped coughing after his RSV hospitalization. Asthma, croup, infections, and reflux would define the next ten years. The mom guilt was gut-wrenching. Look at the consequences of my decision to put my newborn son into daycare. To this day, that decision haunts me.

The next few years were relentless and exhausting. Asher was continuously sick with breathing problems and infections. I also noticed he wasn't developing words or talking. He needed my help. More support than two hours after my work day.

Meanwhile, my job demands kept accelerating. In addition to treating clinic patients, I kept taking on new projects. I agreed to edit a multiple sclerosis book, assist with clinical studies, give presentations, teach residents, and on and on. The workload felt like it was growing each week; it was crushing me. I just couldn't say the word "no".

The wake-up call

I started waking up in the morning with gnawing stomach pain. I tried over-the-counter medicine, antacids, omeprazole, and other treatments for stomach distress. They didn't help much. The pain was bearable. Tony Robbins's words echoed in my head, "I can do this because I have to." I ignored the symptoms.

As weeks passed, the pain lasted longer, became stronger. I continued to push myself as so many parents do, without thinking. I just moved on autopilot. Work all day, take care of an emerging toddler all night. The weight and worry over Asher's medical and developmental issues grew heavier on me. My impressive denial of reality was about to become undeniable.

The reconciliation

On a spring morning in May, I was getting ready for another busy day in the clinic. Outside, it was a gray and gloomy morning—a typical spring day for Seattle. Light rainfall cascaded down the windows. As I stood in the shower, I took a sip of coffee. Yes, I sip my morning coffee while in the shower. Suddenly, a wave of dizziness came over me. I reached for the wall and steadied myself. I took a deep breath and the dizziness passed. Maybe it was the coffee.

I felt a little off, but was certain the feeling would pass. Maybe I was dehydrated from the long day before. Maybe I was dehydrated from drinking coffee first thing in the morning. I headed downstairs and made another cup of coffee for the road. Seattle has the best coffee.

I arrived at the clinic, expecting a typical day. My colleagues were already hard at work in their offices. The architectural design team misunderstood our direction when building the clinic and made the provider offices with clear glass walls that made them into fishbowls. Meanwhile, the conference room had the privacy coating meant for the offices. I waved at my colleagues as I walked past these rooms, hurrying to my office. They laughed lightly, as I arrived about one minute before my first patient was scheduled. Mornings have never been my favorite time of day. Thus, the immediate coffee intake during my morning shower.

Most of the patients on my schedule were women with multiple sclerosis. MS disproportionately affects young women and frequently presents in their twenties, when they are working their way through college or starting a family. When MS strikes, it may cause leg weakness and loss of coordination, making walking difficult. Or the disease may lead to changes in thinking that worsen memory and attention. Treatments were improving though, and at this time, we were more able than ever to stop or slow disease progression.

That day, a physical therapy student was scheduled to work with me. At an academic medical center, teaching and research were part of the day's schedule.

As I briefed the student on the first patient, the wave of dizziness returned. I stumbled. This time, the symptom was joined by stabbing stomach pain. Like I was being stabbed and my attacker just kept turning the knife inside of me. I grimaced and politely excused myself.

Feeling confused, I discreetly walked across the hospital parking lot to the conveniently located emergency room. Working at a medical center had its advantages. After a quick check-in, I was brought to an exam room. The knife continued to twist inside of me. Nausea intensified until I threw up. The doctor examined my stomach, found nothing notable. He ordered labs, all normal. He checked an x-ray; it looked good.

With a puzzled face, the ER doctor stated, "Everything looks ok."

"Really?" I replied. I felt really horrible for someone who was "ok."

I inquired further, "I don't have a pheochromocytoma?" I had been working on a list of all the possible problems for the cause of my stomach pain. Given its severity in spite of my normal abdomen examination, I determined I must have a pheochromocytoma, an exceptionally rare adrenaline-secreting tumor.

"Nope," the doctor replied. "Urine tests for pheo were normal."

"Huh, everything was normal…" I was stunned. I felt like I was dying, but everything showed up as normal. I didn't recall reading this case study in medical school.

The doctor was not sure of the cause of my stomach pain, but didn't find anything concerning. I had learned through the years that this statement is doctor's talk for, "You don't need an operation or an antibiotic, so you can go home now."

So, I went home.

Although there were no clear answers from the medical tests, I knew something was not ok. Despite what the ER doctor said, my body was making it quite clear that it was not ok.

Over the next few weeks, the stabbing stomach pain came and went, seemingly at random. There was no pattern to its onset, no way I could predict when the horrible attack would start or stop. The pain would slowly build up over hours until I threw up. Then, the cycle started all over again. I lost 20 pounds. My eyes sunk in. I could not eat. I could tolerate lemon Gatorade, but that was the extent of my intake. Something was absolutely, definitely, and undeniably not ok.

I took some time off work to rest. Day after day, I sat in our dark house. It was really my husband's house. Painted in a dark brown purplish taupe by the previous owner, the house's interior was cave-like. Even during a sunbreak. Every surface was painted in this dark taupe. The walls, the ceiling, even the cabinets were dark taupe, even the carpet matched. Who WERE these people, the Addams Family? I never understood the paint color choice. I could see the color as an accent wall, but everywhere?

As the days passed, I stared at the walls, the ugly taupe walls. During this heart-wrenching time, I hated the color even more. I decided that as soon as I felt better, those dismal walls were getting a new, vibrant color. Better yet, I was getting out of this house. I would get a house with windows. A light, bright, house. As I stared at my surroundings, the knife twisted again, the pain was unbearable. How could nothing being wrong hurt so much? I questioned myself. I questioned the doctor. I questioned the entire medical testing process.

Nothing was ok

Time would reveal that long-standing, overwhelming, and unrelenting stress provoked a very real disorder. My mom prompted the diagnosis. As I told her what was happening, she remarked, "sounds like you're overwhelmed".

That is when I made the connection; I was having panic attacks. Like many disorders of the brain, it was invisible from the outside and not detectable through medical tests. My panic attacks showed up as severe stomach pain. I never would have thought that stomach pain was the sign of a panic attack! Apparently, the ER doctor didn't know either.

The pain went on for hours at a time, despite the medical literature claiming the attacks typically last 20 minutes or so. I asked my provider about this discrepancy. She shrugged, "Your body doesn't read the textbooks." I felt lucky to have a primary care provider who listened and believed me.

My nervous system had short-circuited due to my stress levels. I had no awareness that I was pushing my limits too hard for too long beyond my capabilities. I didn't listen to my body. So, my brain sent a clear message to my stomach to let me know. A reset of my entire life followed.

Did I fail everyone?

Because of my poor health, I let down my family, my patients, and my work colleagues. I wasn't particularly thrilled with myself either.

After two months, I returned to work on a part-time basis. I was fragile and shaken. Some colleagues did not recognize me. I was gaunt from the rapid weight loss. My denial crumbled under the weight of reality. My situation was not sustainable, it was not healthy. I couldn't live two hours from work, do a good job as a medical director, doctor, researcher, and teacher, and also properly care for my son with additional needs.

Time had revealed that my precious nugget was neurodivergent, meaning Asher's wiring or how his brain worked, was different than what is considered "typical." He processed information and the environment differently. And I needed to figure that out, too.

I could not continue on this unhealthy path. My career and family demands needed to add up to 100 percent of my capability. I needed to get the math right.

Turns out, I had limits. Did Tony Robbins lie to me? Had I taken his words out of context, oversimplified them, and interpreted them to mean what I wanted?

The WHY

Over the next few years, I studied stress-related disorders (SRD). I noticed many of the conditions I had treated—such as chronic back pain, headaches, and digestive issues (with largely normal medical tests)—were rooted in stress, trauma, and feeling constantly overwhelmed. They shared similar elements and followed similar patterns. Recent research has revealed these disorders share a type of problem in the nervous system, too, called nerve sensitization and are referred to as central sensitization syndromes (CSS).

My personal experience was eye-opening and humbling; more importantly, it shed light on how common and disabling stress-related disorders are. Especially stress-related disorders that are not obviously related to stress, like headaches, back pain, and digestive issues. And those that are, such as anxiety disorders and depression. Stress is associated with more than just an increased risk of heart disease and heart attacks.

My experience highlighted the importance of catching SRD in the early stages, being aware of the warning signs, and listening to them. The importance of truly addressing overwhelming stress—burnout level stress—to properly treat these conditions.

" NOT JUST SAYING "REDUCING STRESS" BUT " MAKING AN ACTIONABLE PLAN.

My nervous system is ninety percent healed from my SRD. Had I listened to my body earlier on, when it gave me warning signs, I don't think I would have developed it in the first place. Although I have improved, I never returned to my baseline abilities. Learn from my mistakes.

I hope this book elevates awareness of stress-related disorders of the nervous system so they may be identified earlier and treated proactively. Intervention before the nervous system meltdown, before an emergency room visit, and before a disabling medical condition develops. Early intervention reduces the damaging changes that happen in the brain and nerves when the root issue is not addressed.

Preventing disability that does not need to be is the goal. The majority of the people I treated with stress-related disorders never fully recovered. They did not return to a symptom-free baseline. They were left with recurrent symptoms or the need for daily medications. They were left with a chronic medical condition that affects their daily life. Once something is broken in the body, it seldom returns to 100 percent of the pre-injury level. Kind of like when you sprain your ankle and it never feels as strong or stable as before. Similarly, once a stress-related disorder is triggered, it is hard to fix the broken circuit. The disorder may improve, but long-lasting residual damage persists.

Throughout *Sunbreak*, I present common stress-related disorders through the stories of those who lived them. I share the process and tools I found helpful in healing myself and others. Tools that help build awareness, strengthen the mind-body connection and identify and reduce triggers. And the medical therapies that can help. Ultimately, this process reduces symptoms, reduces suffering, and enables you to take back control of your health and your life.

CHAPTER 3

Stress-related disorders that are not obviously related to stress

CENTRAL SENSITIZATION SYNDROMES (CSS) ARE stress-related disorders and affect upwards of 30 million adults in the United States.[1] They are a common reason for chronic pain. And a common reason people seek out opioids. Yet, in my experience, the root cause or driver of these disorders is rarely addressed in mainstream medical clinics. To bridge this gap in the healthcare system, I will talk about them here.

Let's review the role of stress on performance. I promise to be brief.

The Yerkes-Dodson curve shows the relationship between stress and performance. Mild or even moderate levels of stress actually enhance performance. It's a good stress—yes, there is such a thing! That's when you are motivated and focused.

When the stress level keeps escalating, you hit unmanageable levels that lead to overload and burnout, the dreaded red zone. Here is where you reach distress, exhaustion, anxiety, anger, or a combination of these stress-related states.

---

[1] Muhammad B. Yunus, "Editorial Review (Thematic Issue: An Update on Central Sensitivity Syndromes and the Issues of Nosology and Psychobiology)," Current Rheumatology Reviews 11, no. 2 (July 2015): 70–85. https://doi.org/10.2174/1573397111102150702112236.

THE RELATIONSHIP BETWEEN STRESS AND PERFORMANCE

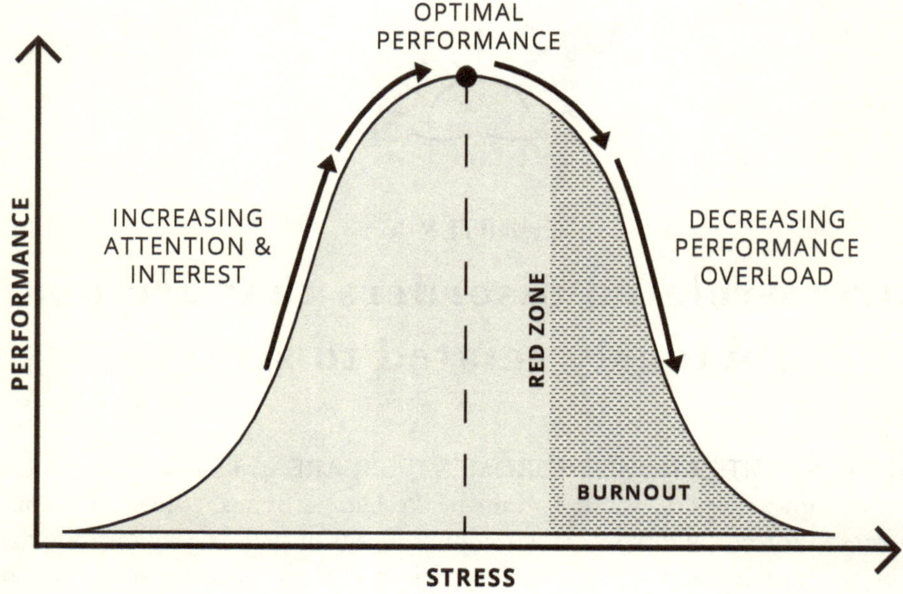

During my clinical practice, I observed that people who were living in the red zone developed one or more of a variety of stress-related disorders (SRD):

- Disabling headaches

- Miserable back pain

- Embarrassing digestive issues

- Crippling anxiety

- Debilitating panic attacks

- Life-threatening depression

Having experienced my own red zone condition that either puzzled providers or was not worth their time, I decided to take a deeper look at the underlying cause of these disorders.

 WHEN YOU ARE LIVING IN THE RED ZONE, THE BODY'S WEAKEST LINK IS BOUND TO BREAK. 

The link between stress and health problems

Between my research and observations, I found long-term, overwhelming stress provokes dysfunction in the nervous system which results in a variety of medical disorders. I witnessed numerous people develop one or more of these disorders while under high stress. Their bodies snapped and broke under unmanageable demands. Like a bridge carrying too much weight for too long. At first, cracks develop. If the weight continues, the structure buckles under the pressure.

Headaches, back pain, and digestive issues may not appear to be stress-related. In fact, stress instigates changes in your physiology, like revving an engine and pushing it to the limits. Then, it feeds more intensely and deeply, creating disorders. You may feel the symptoms in your stomach or back, but the problem may reside in the nervous system. An issue with how the nervous system is relaying pain signals. If the stress and nervous system dysfunction are not addressed, you won't get better. It is like sweeping the garage while intending to clean the kitchen. You have to do the work in the correct room.

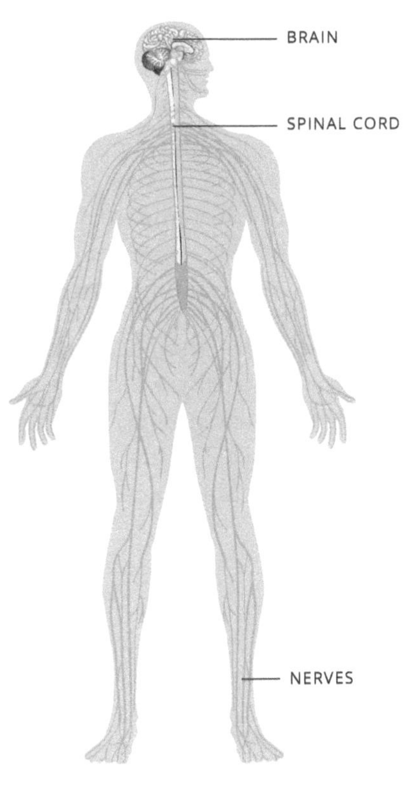

NERVOUS SYSTEM

To better understand how things go wrong in the nervous system, let's review its parts. The nervous system is comprised of the brain, spinal cord, and nerves that control the functions of our body from our thoughts to our movement. When there is dysfunction in the nervous system, it affects the whole body. From your head to your toes. How you feel pain to how energized you are. Left untreated and unmanaged, stress spurs dysfunction in this system.

The onslaught of referrals

As a physical medicine and rehabilitation doctor, my clinic was a funnel for stress-related disorders. Once the traditional medications or procedures failed to help, people were referred to me for symptom management, which meant caring for pain and problems for which their doctors had no course of treatment. These people often shared the same patterns:

- They had disabling symptoms with medical tests that were mostly normal. A mismatch with severe symptoms but normal or only mildly abnormal diagnostic tests.

- These patients were desperate for help and felt their providers thought their symptoms were all in their head.

- They had seen multiple providers with no answers and had undergone multiple procedures that did not help or worsened their symptoms.

The most common referral during my general practice was people with chronic severe back pain without a clear explanation for the intensity of their symptoms. These patients had severe pain, even though their tests showed only mild abnormalities. For example, they had mild arthritis in their lower back, but they were unable to work due to the pain level. Standard care—such as physical therapy, anti-inflammatory medications, and injections—had resulted in minimal benefit. Procedures or surgeries worsened symptoms. Their providers were puzzled at best and dismissive at worst.

These patients feared a serious medical issue had been overlooked or that they imagined their distress. It felt horribly real to them, but when tests showed no reason for their misery, they questioned themselves. "Is it possible what I'm feeling isn't real?" How could something hurt so much and nothing be wrong? I could relate to their painful dilemma.

BOTTOM LINE

Many factors contribute to the development of neurologic conditions, sensitization syndromes, and mental health conditions. Not every case is stress-induced. Not every case has sensitization features. That said, I witnessed how long-term, high stress triggered and worsened these disorders. And how these disorders improved with reduced stress. I not only saw this in the clinic but in family members, friends, work colleagues, and myself. If you're living a high-stress life and experiencing chronic pain, look closely for nerve sensitization.

CHAPTER 4

Melissa's story: Stress strikes in the back

SWEET MELISSA WORKED AS A bartender at a dive bar in small-town Wisconsin. The 34-year-old's nickname was bestowed upon her by the bar patrons. Standing a mere five-foot-two, Melissa had no problem putting a six-foot, 250-pound drunk and disorderly patron in their place. And she could out-drink every last one of them. It was a local bar where the regulars had come for years and everyone knew Melissa. She served up lots of Miller beer and decent burgers. When a customer made a special request, the tough-talker shouted back, "It's not Burger King. You don't get it your way!" The other customers waited for it! Sweet Melissa.

Eventually, Melissa became too good at out-drinking the regulars. Her drinking had become a problem and working in a bar was not going to help her any. She transitioned to an entirely different line of work. She opened Sweet Melissa's makeup station, applying bridal and event makeup. She spent hours each day standing and leaning slightly forward to apply eyeliner and blend eyeshadow. Blending is essential. Standing and leaning in this way, although great for makeup application, is brutal on the back. This position heavily loads the back bones and discs, placing them at increased risk for injury.

Which is what happened next.

Melissa began experiencing a persistent ache in her low back. As the days went by, the discomfort increased. She saw her doctor who assured her it was just a back strain. She tried sitting more at work but the pain persisted. Melissa's doctor then referred her to physical therapy. Weeks later, the pain continued.

In fact, it worsened and spread to a larger area across her back. She tried anti-inflammatory medications like ibuprofen with minimal relief.

Melissa's x-rays showed mild arthritis. Her exam was mostly normal. She experienced sensitivity to touch and discomfort when bending forward and extending. Her strength and walking ability appeared normal. The exam and imaging findings did not explain the severity of Melissa's symptoms. She suffered severe pain and reduced function but nothing in her medical tests offered a physical reason for her symptoms. Mild arthritis is not typically disabling. A back strain should have healed after a few weeks.

Melissa cut back her work hours. She couldn't stand or sit all day anymore. She needed to change positions constantly. And the physical strain and pain exhausted her. She needed more rest.

Given her continued decline, Melissa's doctor ordered a back MRI. It showed mild degenerative disc disease. As serious as that sounds, it is the medical term for arthritis in the spine, and the doctor described it as "mild", according to the MRI. Arthritis changes in the back are common in people by their 30s and 40s, so these results were not all that helpful. Many people with these MRI findings have no symptoms at all. Nonetheless, she received a round of epidural spinal injections to reduce the pain, "just in case" they might help. They didn't.

Spine treatment is not as straightforward as other joints, like the knee or hip where the treatments are more predictable and generally work well. The spine is a complex puzzle with numerous pain generators. The pain can arise from muscles, bones, discs, or nerves. The pain can also arise from within the nervous system—the brain, which is the part of the body that processes pain signals.

Two years, with no answer

For the next two years, Melissa moved as little as possible because she was afraid the pain would get worse. Then the weight came on. Her depression worsened. She was without hope and feared this depressing situation was her new life.

During this time, the four or five doctors Melissa saw didn't seem to know about sensitization and how stress contributed to her health problems. The same standard approach of physical therapy, ibuprofen, and injections was recommended time and time again. The results were similar to the previous three trials.

Melissa was afraid doctors thought she was seeking drugs. And they confirmed her suspicion. It took six doctor visits or more at a medical clinic before the staff trusted Melissa wasn't just there for drugs. That she desperately wanted help. That she was searching for answers. Trying to understand why the standard treatments did not work for her. She did ask for opioids at one point but not because she was trying to get high but because she was desperate for relief and it was all she knew that might help. Melissa wasn't seeking drugs. She was seeking relief.

Melissa felt shamed by some of the medical staff at the clinic. When she called the clinic with questions, she was greeted with a condescending tone. She recalled one particularly hard day when she called the clinic with a question and the staff's response was, "Aren't you on enough medicine? What else do you want?"

Doubt, guilt, depression, and addiction

The struggle wasn't just in the clinic, but also in the people around her. Co-workers, friends, and family were annoyed by Melissa's pain issues.

She was ridiculed, judged, and lectured because they didn't think anything was clinically wrong. She looked ok and her medical tests were mostly normal. Based on their understanding of pain, she was exaggerating or faking.

Melissa felt guilty that she couldn't do anything. Guilty that she couldn't play with her kids because she didn't have the energy. Guilty for how much her parents helped, since she no longer worked. She felt she was wasting her life, but unable to do anything about it. She felt worthless, a burden to everyone around her.

The only relief Melissa knew came from opioid pain medication. At this point, she had become dependent on pain medication. She understood that the amount of opioid she needed to dull the pain was that of a person dying of cancer. Despite the high dose of pain medication, she was still not functioning. She couldn't work and struggled to take care of her kids. Melissa had to retrain her brain that medications weren't the only answer.

Missed cause of misery–nerve sensitization

After a couple of years of physical and emotional suffering, Melissa was referred to a specialist who understood nerve sensitization. She saw Melissa's pain and disability were much greater than expected given her physical exam and imaging findings. Melissa had system-wide symptoms, including brain fog and debilitating fatigue. She struggled to sleep at night. She hadn't mentioned these non-pain symptoms to her previous providers because she didn't realize they were related. The non-pain symptoms were a clue of system-wide dysfunction, nerve sensitization.

Melissa's misery had started with a minor back injury, too much strain on her back from leaning over eight hours a day applying makeup. But the initial injury no longer explained the growing pain and disability. The time required to heal a back strain or calm an arthritis flare had long since passed. Her pain was no longer solely a muscle or joint issue. Another process had been triggered. There was now dysfunction in the nervous system, too. A problem with how pain signals are processed. And, unfortunately, this problem could not be seen or measured on standard medical tests. You can't see a sensitized nerve on an MRI or x-ray, even though it's there.

Melissa's symptoms were the end expression of multiple issues that came together for a "perfect storm" of chronic pain:

- Mild back arthritis and muscle strain

- Nerve sensitization

- Overwhelming stress

The progression from mild to severe

Here is how sensitization turns a mild issue into a disabling condition:

1. Melissa started with moderate discomfort from a back injury.

2. The injury triggered nerve sensitization.

3. Sensitization amplified the pain signals, making every movement, every activity, hurt severely. She felt more pain more severely than someone who has back arthritis but without sensitization.

Two separate health conditions—arthritis and nerve sensitization. But can you see how, when they connect, the pain becomes more intense? It's like two wires sparking when they touch one another.

Depression and addiction also played a role in Melissa's condition. Negative emotions intensify pain. Meanwhile, Melissa's desperate search for relief brought her to opioids and resulted in addiction. The combination of factors contributed to her disability—arthritis, nerve sensitization, depression, and addiction. No factor was solely to blame.

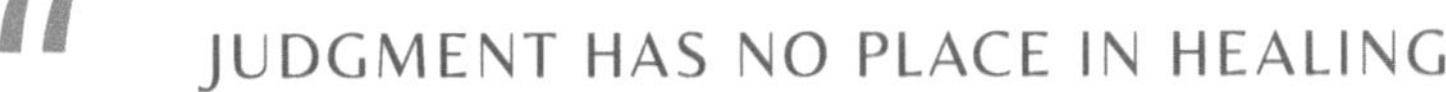 

JUDGMENT HAS NO PLACE IN HEALING.

To understand how all the different factors contributed to her symptoms, think of it this way. Let's say, Melissa's total pain score is a ten out of ten (10/10). Her back arthritis causes two pain points. Sensitization causes four pain points. Depression adds two pain points. When she is under overwhelming stress that adds another two pain points, giving her a ten out of ten pain level. In her case, most of the dysfunction causing pain was within the nervous system. A spinal injection or back surgery is not going to help because the problem is in the nervous system.

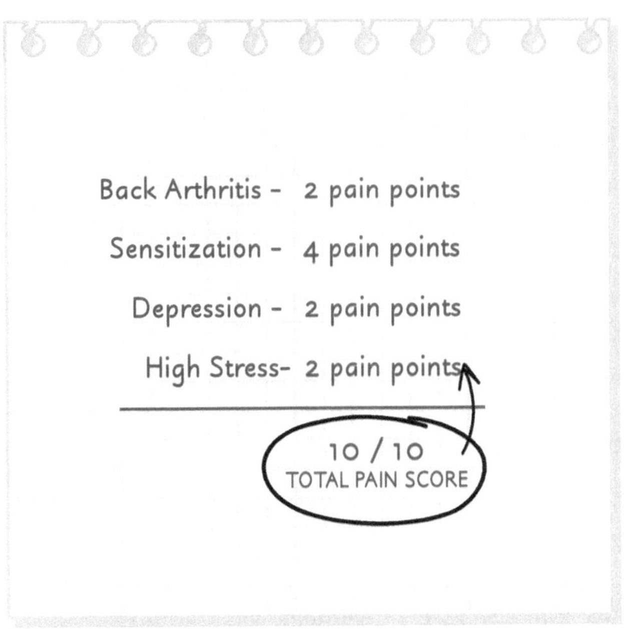

Eventually, Melissa started to improve when she understood the factors contributing to her symptoms. The knowledge helped her take action rather than feel hopeless.

The road to wellness starts with knowledge

Melissa's path to recovery consisted of:

1. Understanding how sensitization affects pain levels

2. Managing medications

3. Building awareness of the stress-body connection

4. Following an exercise program of her choosing

5. Connecting to a caring and supportive community

The role of sensitization in pain levels. Becoming aware of sensitization's effects on her body gave Melissa the power to improve her situation. When she understood that her symptoms were related to sensitization rather than a worsening injury, she no longer feared moving. Knowledge put Melissa in a better mindset to manage the symptoms.

The right medicines. Medication management shifted to the types that work for nerve sensitization and nerve pain—medications that calm the over-reactive nerves. Ibuprofen is the wrong type for relieving nerve or sensitization pain, so it's ineffective.

Stress reduction and self-care. Melissa became aware of how stress worsened her back symptoms. This awareness empowered her to reduce stress. She recognized the importance of self-care. She couldn't take care of her kids if she was not well. She became ok with making her needs a priority, rather than something that can be blown off.

Emotional support and exercise. She joined a gym, which gave her a sense of community. Melissa surrounded herself with people vested in her getting healthy. She made like-minded friends of all ages. Her back felt better with regular workouts. She realized movement was the answer, not the enemy. She lost weight and felt good.

Melissa's mental health improved when she regained hope. She understood her struggles were real, that she wasn't imagining them as all her coworkers, family, and many providers believed. At last, she had proof that she wasn't just crazy or being overly dramatic. This validation rescued her from the depths of despair. She finally had a course of real treatment, providing real help.

> **" AS SIMPLE AS IT SOUNDS, BECOMING AWARE OF SENSITIZATION AND STRESS EFFECTS ON HER BODY GAVE MELISSA THE POWER TO IMPROVE HER SITUATION. "**

After twelve months of sticking to this program, Melissa regained her health, wellness, and happiness. Recovery is a process that takes time. To this day, Melissa is relieved the pain is better and thankful to have discovered the values of fitness and health at a much deeper level. She does still use medications, but she functions now. She cares for her kids and has a part-time house painting business. She enjoys the movement and artistry that comes with painting.

Melissa regained control of her life and health. Knowledge is power when managing this type of disorder.

CHAPTER 5

Nerves gone rogue: Sensitization syndromes

MELISSA'S CHRONIC BACK PAIN RESULTED from arthritis and nerve sensitization. The arthritis did not cause that much discomfort but when you add in the nerve sensitization, it becomes disabling. Chronic back pain belongs to the group of medical conditions called central sensitization syndromes (CSS). Other examples include chronic migraine, irritable bowel, and chronic bladder pain. The individual conditions differ in many ways but all share the feature of over-reactive nerves (sensitization).

High stress is one of the triggers for sensitization syndromes. The symptoms also worsen or flare with stress.

Everyone's body is a little different and communicates with them in its own way. Some people develop headaches, some get stomachaches, while others experience flares of pain in the back.

The common sensitization syndromes I saw are listed below.

Body System	Sensitization Syndrome
Joints/muscles	Chronic back pain and neck pain
	Chronic muscle pain (myofascial pain syndrome)
	Fibromyalgia
	Temporomandibular joint disorder

Digestive	Chronic heartburn
	Stomach pain
	Irritable bowel syndrome
Neurologic	Migraine headaches
	Chronic tension-type headaches
Urinary	Chronic bladder pain (i.e., interstitial cystitis)
Reproductive	Chronic pelvic pain

There is a good chance you or someone you know suffers from a central sensitization syndrome. Someone with chronic migraines for years? Someone with chronic back pain for years? Someone with chronic digestive symptoms for years? Years of severe symptoms without an adequate explanation? These are all potential cases of sensitization. I have a family member with chronic headaches, another with chronic back pain, one friend with chronic bladder pain, and another with irritable bowel syndrome! And these are just people I know closely. Everywhere I look, whether it is in my clinic or in my circle of friends and family, I see people struggling with these conditions and struggling to find care for them. If you or someone you know is suffering with CSS, please tell them there is help. This book is a resource to find answers and help that is not widely available in the current healthcare system.

You've got a lot of nerve

Nerve sensitization arises from abnormalities in how pain signals are processed and perceived in the brain, spinal cord, and nerves. Sensitization makes the nerves more sensitive and more reactive to stimuli which increases pain levels. There is increased reactivity to normal sensory inputs, such as touch and movement.[2]

Sensitized nerves exaggerate the pain signal when reporting it to the brain. The reactive nerves send more pain signals, more often. They are like tattletales, constantly telling the brain something is wrong. The person then perceives something serious is wrong. It's what I call a "maladaptive biologic process". The nerves get confused and adjust in an unhelpful way; the brain believes the tattletale nerves. This is why Melissa was so impaired from her mild arthritis.

---

[2] Jo Nijs et al., "Nociplastic Pain Criteria or Recognition of Central Sensitization? Pain Phenotyping in the Past, Present and Future," Journal of Clinical Medicine 10, no. 15 (July 21, 2021): 3203. https://doi.org/10.3390/jcm10153203.

The tattletales exaggerated the injury level and told her brain it was severe. Her nerves had gone rogue.

How sensitization creates misery

When sensitization is present, it changes how you experience pain. You feel it more easily, more intensely, and in more places.

Here are the three ways that sensitization exaggerates pain levels.

1. Pain hypersensitivity is increased sensitivity to sensory inputs, such as touch, pressure, and movement. For example, let's look at two people, one with sensitization and the other without it. They both lift a 50-pound box and feel a pull in the back. The person without sensitization reports the pain as a "three out of ten". Meanwhile, the person with sensitization reports the pain as a "seven out of ten". The nerves are telling the brain it hurts more than what a person without the condition feels. It's not the person overreacting; the intensity is very real. The sensation is because the nerves are hypersensitive.

2. Pain in response to things that aren't normally painful. Light pressure on the back muscles shouldn't cause discomfort outside of an injury. With nerve sensitization, a mild touch can prompt a substantial pain response. And, after being touched, there can be unpleasant sensations, like burning or tingling. Your partner reaches over to rub your back and you jerk away; the light touch is painful instead of comforting. Your partner may feel rebuffed, thinking you're overreacting. But you know that you're not.

3. The pain spreads to more parts of the body. With sensitization, pain spreads beyond the injured area, such as the joint or nerve. One example is with back pain. Instead of a small area of the back hurting, a person with nerve sensitization may feel pain across the back and down into the thighs. Another example is with nerves, someone with a pinched nerve may feel their entire leg is numb, instead of just the area supplied by the irritated nerve.

Non-pain symptoms still hurt

In addition to affecting how pain is experienced, sensitization causes symptoms that affect the entire body. Called "non-pain symptoms", they include activity limiting fatigue, disrupted sleep, and thinking difficulties. Tattletale nerves throw the entire nervous system off, like a malfunctioning electrical panel. The electricity doesn't flow right and the system sends incorrect signals.

The **fatigue** can be severe with a much lower energy level compared to others of the same age and health. Fatigue sets in much sooner and recovery lasts longer. For example, after an hour of intense exercise, someone with sensitization may need to rest for the remainder of the day or two days. If you recall Melissa, her fatigue limited her ability to care for and play with her kids. It was one of her most troubling symptoms.

Sleep issues range from frequently waking up at night to feeling tired and unrefreshed in the morning—when you should feel most rested. Compounding the struggle, poor sleep increases pain sensitivity and worsens fatigue. Your abilities plummet with poor sleep.

Brain fog is another issue. With brain fog, the mind feels muddled and slow. Memory is poor and it's hard to concentrate. You get to work and try focusing on your task list but it takes forever because you can't think clearly.

The environment is full of sensory inputs and nerve sensitization magnifies these stimuli, too. The impact of harsh lights, loud noise, and odors is amplified. These stimuli may provoke headaches, nausea, or dizziness.

Taken together, the symptoms cause fatigue and disrupted sleep which limits activities. Then brain fog makes it harder to get through the activities. Now add sensitivity to light, noise, and smells making you uncomfortable. Combined, the non-pain symptoms may limit you more than the pain!

Between the pain condition—such as headaches or back pain—and the non-pain symptoms, nerve sensitization affects the function of the entire body. Your brain and nervous system are in charge of helping you think clearly, be active, and regulate sleep. If that system is not working normally, all its functions are affected. With sensitization syndromes, the disorder does not stem from just the back or head or stomach, but from the entire nervous system. That is how chronic back pain or irritable bowel can be paired with brain fog, sleep troubles, and fatigue.

BOTTOM LINE

Central sensitization syndromes are the most frequent type of stress-related disorder I encounter. When people don't respond to standard therapy—like physical therapy or anti-inflammatory medications—stress or sensitization is the missing piece that needs to be addressed. If sensitization is the main driver of symptoms, the treatment requires a different approach.

CHAPTER 6

Why living in the stress response makes you sick

"If you are a zebra running for your life, or a lion sprinting for your meal, your body's physiological response mechanisms are superbly adapted for dealing with such short-term physical emergencies. For the vast majority of beasts on this planet, stress is about a short-term crisis, after which it's either over with or you're over with. When we sit around and worry about stressful things, we turn on the same physiological responses—but they are potentially a disaster when provoked chronically. A large body of evidence suggests that stress-related disease emerges, predominantly, out of the fact we so often activate a physiological system that has evolved for responding to acute physical emergencies, but we turn it on for months on end, worrying about mortgages, relationships, and promotions."

—Robert M. Sapolsky
Why Zebras Don't Get Ulcers[3]

HOW THE STRESS RESPONSE WORKS. Revered scientist Robert Sapolsky wrote one of the most, if not the most, prominent books on how stress affects the body in *Why Zebras Don't Get Ulcers*. Robert Sapolsky is like the Brad Pitt of the physiology world. Physiology and medical students fawn over his intellectual acumen and his riveting lectures. Screaming outside a lecture hall just to get a glimpse of him. Well, not really, but I feel that way on the inside when I listen to his physiology lectures on YouTube.

---

[3] Robert M. Sapolsky, *Why Zebras Don't Get Ulcers: The Acclaimed Guide to Stress, Stress-Related Diseases, and Coping - Now Revised and Updated* (Holt Paperbacks, 2004).

In his book, Sapolsky explains in extraordinary detail how stress adversely affects each body system, from the heart to reproduction. He explains the changes in how the body works during stress physiology and why they increase the risk for medical conditions. His work lays the foundation for understanding and managing stress-related disorders.

How stress, and in particular chronic stress, affects the body is through the stress response. The response is also termed the fight-or-flight response. Or in my case, more of a "freeze" response, because I tend to freeze during an emergency. I would have been a horrible emergency room physician. Anyway, the body mounts a stress response to any perceived threat. Or any thought of a perceived threat.

From an evolutionary standpoint, this response developed to improve survival from an immediate physical threat. For instance, you are walking on a remote trail in the mountains and hear something bustling in the trees. The sound creeps closer. You scan the area, then freeze as a bear steps onto the trail and stares into your eyes.

The stress response has just been activated. The body starts secreting stress hormones, including cortisol and adrenaline. Stress hormones surge through the body, making the heart beat faster and increasing blood flow to muscles. Heart rate, blood pressure, and breathing rate increase to get energy (glucose) and oxygen to muscles quickly so they can react faster. This enhances physical prowess and chances of survival. You can fight harder or flee faster.

Meanwhile, processes like digestion, growth, tissue repair, and reproduction are put on hold. All of the body's resources are directed toward the emergency. As Sapolsky explains, "There is no need to digest lunch if you are about to become lunch." If digestion, growth, and repair are put on hold for years due to chronic stress, the risk of developing medical conditions increases.

Over the short term, the stress response is adaptive, it helps the body adjust to the situation to maximize survival. The response was intended to run for short periods of time during physical emergencies. Over the long term, stress physiology breaks the body down. We aren't physiologically designed to handle it for extended periods.

For example, let's look at how the stress response affects the heart. If your blood pressure spikes to 190/110 while you escape from a bear on the trail, that is helpful. The response delivers energy for your muscles to work optimally. If your blood pressure is 190/110 during work all day, every day, that is going to increase your risk of heart disease and dying from a heart attack.

From a metabolic standpoint, chronic stress leads to a higher risk of diabetes. The hormones of the stress response mobilize energy. They cause glucose to pour into the bloodstream and make cells less sensitive to insulin. This process promotes insulin resistance, which is the precursor to diabetes.

The hormones released during the stress response switch on inflammation in the nervous system which increases the risk of developing sensitization syndromes. The inflammation, called neuroinflammation, sets off nerve sensitization and pain conditions.[4]

---

[4] Ru-Rong Ji et al., "Neuroinflammation and Central Sensitization in Chronic and Widespread Pain," Anesthesiology 129, no. 2 (August 1, 2018): 343–66, https://doi.org/10.1097/aln.0000000000002130.

Triggers of the stress response

The stress response does not differentiate between types of stressors. There is not one response for a bear encounter, a response for work stress, and a response for kid stress. The same response is put into effect whether the stress is from a physical threat or from psychological strain.

> WHETHER YOU ARE EYE TO EYE WITH A BEAR OR EYE TO EYE WITH YOUR CHECKBOOK, THE SAME STRESS RESPONSE IS TRIGGERED.

This is problematic since modern-day stress is mostly from psychological strain arising from work demands, financial struggles, and family needs. Unfortunately, regardless of the perceived threat, the body prepares to fight a bear.

Not only is the same stress response activated by physical or psychological stress, but it can also be induced by thoughts alone. Just thinking about work demands or financial struggles starts the stress response. This is one reason therapeutic practices, like mindfulness and meditation, are helpful. They calm the stress response. Mindfulness activities improve control over our thoughts, especially non-productive, negative thoughts. This, in turn, reduces the stress response and harmful stress physiology. Our thoughts have a direct effect on how our body works.

The stress response equips us to escape a threat. With the daily psychological stress that's rampant in today's world, the stress response can be more damaging than the stressors themselves. Running fast won't help you escape a work deadline. Living each day with stress-induced high blood pressure may take you out as fast as the bear, from a heart attack.

CHAPTER 7

Bryan's story: Stress can make your head explode

BRYAN BUILT HIS CONSTRUCTION COMPANY from the ground up. He acted as CEO, COO, HR, and IT. On top of that, he helped with the day-to-day work. He had been working at this pace for ten years. He had just endured six months that had been especially stress-filled. The team was working on a two-year school renovation. The school representative—let's call him Ivan—tortured the team. He demanded changes beyond the scope of the project and then refused to pay for them after Bryan's crew completed the tasks. Ivan was aggressive, arrogant, and, worse, he didn't know what he was talking about. He didn't understand construction. Ivan postured, provoked, and then made demands that didn't make sense. One by one, project managers failed at working with this guy. Bryan had gone through three project managers, each one ending up refusing to work with Ivan and, in one instance, in the emergency room. One employee's hands shook as he talked about Ivan. Another developed chest pain, which turned out to be a stress-induced panic attack. The third just put his hands up and said "I can't, I can't work with him anymore!" It became Bryan's turn to deal with Ivan the Terrible, a public menace on a power trip.

During this six-month stretch, Bryan presented to the clinic urgently with piercing pain behind his left eye. As he talked, his upper eyelid drooped and his eye watered. His nose was congested and running. Since Bryan was afraid he might be dying, we both felt a visit to the emergency room was the safest course of action.

The eye pain continued to increase in intensity to the worst pain Bryan had ever experienced. He arrived at the emergency room, fearing he was having a stroke or a bleeding aneurysm. Upon arrival, he was ushered to the triage area. His blood pressure was high. That could be from pain or from the body increasing blood pressure to push blood to an area with inadequate flow, like from a stroke. Bryan immediately had a CT scan of his head to check for a bleed. The ER was overflowing with patients, so he laid on a stretcher in the hallway waiting for the results. Hour after hour passed. The unrelenting pain continued. Panic and fear grew. Not being a doctor, Bryan didn't know that when it takes forever to get test results, it means the results are normal. Finally, the emergency room doctor emerged with Bryan's results. He was remarkably calm in the midst of the surrounding chaos.

The doctor took a seat next to Bryan to talk with him at eye level. "Your head CT is normal. No bleeding and no other concerning abnormalities. I think this is a migraine headache. I see a fair number of these in guys your age. Let's try a few medications to see if we can calm the headache."

After three hours of the worst pain of his life, Bryan finally had reassurance he was going to be ok, relatively speaking. His body's stress response had been in overdrive for too long. A migraine with autonomic features was triggered. Although the pain calmed with medications, Bryan's headache recurred every day.

Is it a coincidence that stress disorders cause such acute, severe distress that they stop someone in the middle of the day to rush to the emergency room? To the point that they feel they are dying?

For Bryan, a man deeply committed to his work, the severe pain forced him to stop and pay attention. There was nothing normal or ok about the intense pain, the daily recurring headache.

Bryan took the next two weeks off work to rest. His head pain was still a constant five out of ten with spikes of agonizing pain. I started him on a daily headache prevention medication—propranolol, a beta blocker. The headache pain slowly decreased. Beta blockers, the workhorse of cardiology and headache prevention. Luckily, this one worked well.

We discussed the start of his severe headaches that occurred during a period of extremely high stress. I warned Bryan that continuing at that level was unsustainable. The intense stress triggered debilitating autonomic headaches, following years of a charged-up autonomic nervous system ("stress physiology"). His body and his brain were breaking down.

For Bryan, the treatment plan for his stress-related disorder included:

1. Building awareness of the effect of stress on his physical body, communicated through headaches

2. Lowering stress levels

3. Medication

He needed daily headache prevention medication to fight off the headaches. Each time Bryan attempted to wean himself off the medication, the headaches returned. He needed to continue taking them. The long period of unrelenting stress led to a chronic condition.

Over the next few months, Bryan had to figure out how to lower his stress levels at work. Could he afford to hire help? Could he get his nightmare client under control? Did he need to close the business that he spent ten years building?

Bryan was able to hire additional staff to delegate portions of the work and remain in business. The project with Ivan was far enough along that Bryan transitioned the close-out to another employee, distributing the stress of working with Ivan to lessen the impact. Bryan's spouse forbade any further projects involving Ivan. Smart move!

BOTTOM LINE

Bryan's headaches stabilized on preventative medication. When he entered a high-stress period, however, the piercing pain behind his eye crept back. A sharp reminder the stress level was too much.

The nervous system remembers stress and trauma, and tries to shield us from further attack. The human body speaks to us through physical symptoms.

Years later, Bryan continues to run his company. He still needs the daily medication or the headaches return. The cautionary note is that although his headaches improved with lowered stress, they never totally resolved. Bryan now has a chronic headache disorder. The stress level triggered a chronic medical condition that could be managed but not healed.

I've witnessed too many people "mind over matter" into a medical disorder. I don't want you to reach that point. Awareness with early action is the path to wellness. And it starts with educating yourself. If you are already there, living with a chronic disorder, awareness and education helps manage it and reduce symptoms.

CHAPTER 8

How sensitization turns up the pain

WHEN I WAS IN MEDICAL training, the various central sensitization syndromes (CSS) were referred to and treated separately. They affected separate body systems, so the specialist in that body system treated it. There was no relationship seen between someone with a chronic headache disorder and chronic back pain. No relationship between someone with chronic digestive issues and chronic bladder pain. There was no obvious connection between them. We now understand the conditions do have a connection. A connection that is pivotal to proper treatment.

Research shows that these seemingly unrelated conditions share a common underlying problem—sensitization of the nervous system. Sensitization causes the nerves to become more sensitive and reactive to stimuli. More sensitive nerves mean more symptoms, more often. CSS also share the same group of risk factors that lead to their development.

How sensitization starts

If you're reading this book, you might already be experiencing a CSS. But you should understand the factors that increase the risk of developing one.

Stress

Long-term stress is a trigger for sensitization syndromes. The hormones released during the stress response switch on an inflammatory state, which causes inflammation in the nervous system. The inflammation sensitizes the nerves and increases the risk of developing a CSS.

Similarly, high stress worsens symptoms. Recall Bryan and his chronic headaches. His headache disorder developed during an extended period of high stress. Bryan's autonomic system was in overdrive for ten years and spilled over into migraines with autonomic features. His headaches returned each time his stress levels rose too high.

Physical injury

Another important factor in the development of sensitization syndromes is physical injury. For example, Sweet Melissa started with a minor back injury (muscle strain and arthritis flare). Over time, sensitization developed, the pain continued even after the injury healed. An injury to a joint is a common start to sensitization.[5]

Genetics

As with many medical conditions, some people are genetically predisposed to certain ones. Genetics even affect how you experience pain through genes specific to pain sensitivity! If you have a low pain tolerance, your genetics may have wired you that way.

Psychological factors

Sensitization syndromes frequently occur alongside mental health conditions, such as depression and anxiety. Each one affects and worsens the other. The pain disorder increases the risk of depression and anxiety. Anxiety and depression intensify pain from the disorder. A vicious cycle follows. Sometimes, chronic back pain triggers depression. Sometimes, depression intensifies back pain.

The pain and emotion circuits process pain together, increasing pain perception in the brain. Unfortunately, each individual condition negatively affects the other. It is not that you are "just depressed" or "just anxious"; depression and anxiety increase the pain perception.

Trauma

Childhood trauma and abuse are common with certain sensitization syndromes. This topic is worth a book in and of itself. In the clinic, I recall seeing young women present with whole-body pain, fibromyalgia, and chronic bladder pain. More often than not, these individuals suffered sexual abuse or severe trauma

---

[5] Muhammad B. Yunus, "Editorial Review (Thematic Issue: An Update on Central Sensitivity Syndromes and the Issues of Nosology and Psychobiology)," Current Rheumatology Reviews 11, no. 2 (July 2015): 70–85, https://doi.org/10.2174/157339711102150702112 236.

as children, abuse that lasted for years.

Abuse may act as the trigger—the injury—initiating the physical changes that lead to sensitization. For example, women who have suffered sexual abuse develop chronic pain in the bladder or pelvic area, the location of the abuse. The physical trauma causes local inflammation that affects the nerves resulting in neuroinflammation. Emotional trauma and the stress response cause system-wide inflammation. Neuroinflammation then leads to sensitization and chronic pain.

The brain and nervous system become vigilant guard dogs to keep away repeat trauma. The brain is hyper-responsive to any stimuli it fears may be placing it back in harm's way. Trauma gets embedded in the nervous system.

How the pain progresses

Here's how sensitization intensifies pain:

1. Nerve sensitization is a result of dysfunction in the nervous system.

2. Sensitization changes how pain signals are processed and perceived in the brain, spinal cord, and nerves.

3. Abnormal processing of signals results in increased responsiveness to sensory inputs—like touch and movement—as well as increased reactivity to sensory stimuli including light, sound, and smells.[6]

4. The increased sensitivity intensifies pain. Nerves are more reactive. Pain comes on faster and lasts longer.

5. The pain continues, even in the absence of an injury.

The abnormal changes in the nervous system from sensitization do not show-up on standard medical tests. Without "proof" of an injury or other reason for the pain, your provider may not understand why you hurt. Yet, the intensity of the discomfort can make you afraid to move or leave the house. Remember Melissa, she developed a fear of moving, afraid the movement would injure her further.

Current theory on how sensitization develops is that an inciting event—such as an injury, high stress, or trauma—initiates a cascade of inflammation that spreads to the nervous system, resulting in neuroinflammation. Neuroinflam-

---

[6] Jo Nijs et al., "Nociplastic Pain Criteria or Recognition of Central Sensitization? Pain Phenotyping in the Past, Present and Future," Journal of Clinical Medicine 10, no. 15 (July 21, 2021): 3203. https://doi.org/10.3390/jcm10153203.

mation sensitizes the nerves and disrupts normal processing of pain signals.

Think of the brain and nerves like an electrical panel. The panel maintains balance in the system, adjusting its inputs and outputs, creating an even flow of signals throughout the body. Nerve sensitization turns up the signal frequency too high, disrupting the function of the system. The body has more intense incoming pain signals and loses the ability to turn down those signals. The loss of these two critical processes translates to more pain and less protection, which happens at each level of the nervous system.[7]

SENSITIZATION AFFECTS EACH LEVEL OF THE NERVOUS SYSTEM

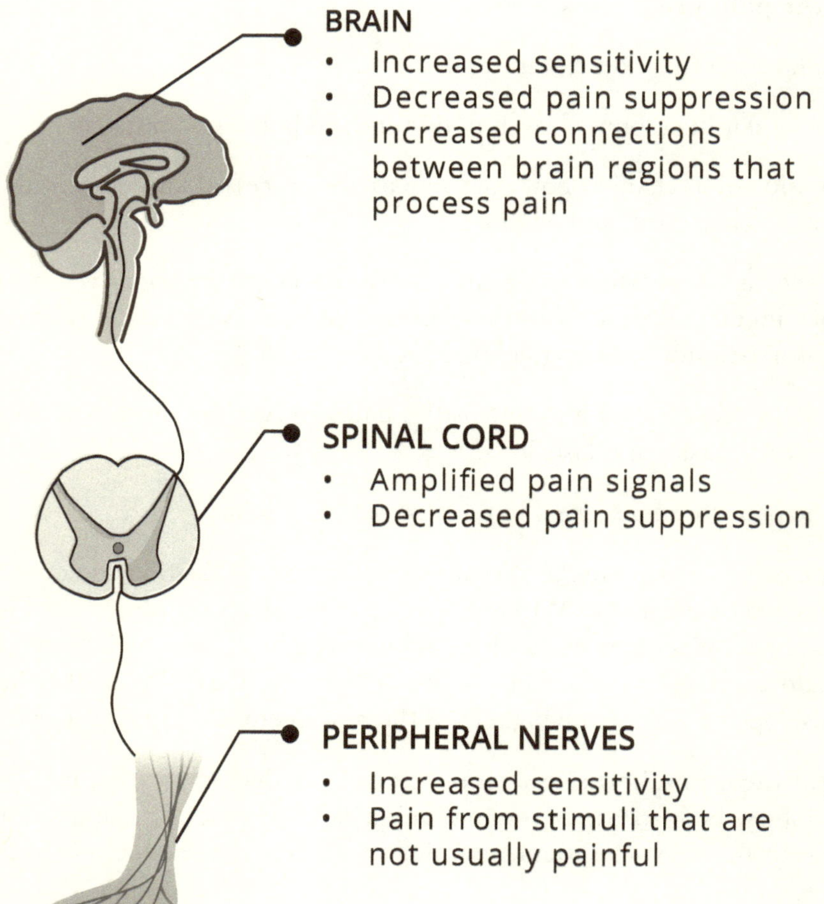

[7] Mary-Ann Fitzcharles et al., "Nociplastic Pain: Towards an Understanding of Prevalent Pain Conditions," The Lancet 397, no. 10289 (May 1, 2021): 2098–2110.

Functional **MRI** is a radiology test that shows what areas of the brain are active during certain tasks, such as picking up objects or feeling pain. It has enabled scientists to see how sensitization changes brain function. At last, visual proof of what is going wrong!

Imaging reveals those with sensitization process pain differently. They have increased connections between brain regions that process pain and decreased activity in areas that suppress pain. They perceive more pain and have less protection from it.

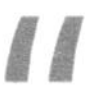

THE ENTIRE ELECTRIC PANEL
MALFUNCTIONS. AT THIS POINT, THE
NERVOUS SYSTEM NEEDS A REBOOT.

BOTTOM LINE

Central sensitization syndromes vary in their symptoms but they all share the feature of nerve sensitization. Sensitization arises from dysfunction in the nervous system. The dysfunction causes more intense pain signals and loss of the body's ability to turn down the pain signals. The balance is lost like a malfunctioning electrical panel. These changes occur at each level of the nervous system, the brain, spinal cord, and nerves. Risk factors that lead to sensitization include stress, injury, genetics, and trauma. Now that functional **MRI** provides a visual of brain function, we can see how sensitization changes the way the brain processes pain.

CHAPTER 9

Olivia's story: Abuse has lifelong impacts

CHILDHOOD TRAUMA AND ABUSE ARE risk factors for chronic bladder pain, pelvic pain, and fibromyalgia. Abuse is a physical and emotional trigger that sets into motion the changes that lead to sensitization syndromes developing.

Olivia came to see me when she was twenty years old, suffering from the pain and misery of chronic and severe bladder pain. She had been diagnosed with interstitial cystitis, a bladder pain condition characterized by urinary urgency, frequency, and pelvic pain. If you've ever had a bladder infection, you can appreciate the intense discomfort. Imagine if your bladder infection pain never went away; that is what living with interstitial cystitis feels like.

Olivia endured bladder pain on a daily basis. During high stress times, the pain spiked to an excruciating level, driving her to the emergency room desperate for relief. Olivia had seen multiple gynecologists, but none of the interventions had helped. She was trying to get through college, but kept experiencing horrible pain episodes that would make her miss days of school or exams. She had never been pregnant or had surgery, so it was unusual for such a young woman to have severe pelvic pain. That was a sign there was more to her story.

In my first visit with Olivia, I didn't want to get too personal too fast. Still, I suspected the underlying issue warranted this difficult conversation and I pushed ahead.

I gently inquired, "Olivia, were you ever abused?"

To my surprise, she quickly responded, "Yes."

I continued, "I am sorry to bring this up, but it may be related to your pelvic pain. Can you tell me what kind of abuse you suffered?"

Olivia replied, "I was sexually abused by a family member from the time I was eight until I was eleven years old."

My heart sank. Three years of sexual abuse by someone she should trust.

"Did you ever get help for this, such as trauma therapy?"

She responded stoically, "No. You are the first person I have told."

We spent the next hour discussing the relationship between her symptoms and her early life trauma. I explained to Olivia that abuse acts as a trigger, an injury, that puts in motion the physical changes that lead to sensitization. The physical trauma causes inflammation in the abused area. The psychological stress induces low level inflammation in the body as well. The inflammation affects the nerves leading to neuroinflammation. The inflammation sensitizes the nerves leading to a chronic pain condition.

As I listened, I saw the painful memories rush back to her. As a woman and a physician, I wanted to get her the right help. I connected Olivia to a specialty clinic that helps sexual abuse victims and provides trauma therapy. We discussed treatment that would help her physically. I could lower her pain level, make it more manageable, while she worked through healing.

The physical repercussions of abuse

Chronic bladder pain, like Olivia's, is often associated with a history of abuse. A study of women with interstitial cystitis found that 49 percent reported a history of abuse.[8] Of those reporting abuse, 92 percent reported emotional abuse, 78 percent reported physical abuse, and 68 percent reported sexual abuse. Those numbers represent a much higher prevalence of abuse than reported in the general population. In my personal experience with women patients, the abuse rate is more like 80 percent. It just isn't reported ... for so many reasons.

---

[8] Kenneth M. Peters et al., "Fact or Fiction—Is Abuse Prevalent in Patients With Interstitial Cystitis? Results From a Community Survey and Clinic Population," The Journal of Urology 178, no. 3 (September 2007): 891–95. https://doi.org/10.1016/j.juro.2007.05.047.

In addition to fibromyalgia, bladder pain, and pelvic pain, early life adversity and trauma are also risk factors for headaches, irritable bowel, and TMJ.[9] Adversity encompasses various types of situations, from poor parent-to-parent and parent-to-child relationships, physical abuse, and sexual abuse.

> **" PEOPLE WHO SUFFER SEVERE TRAUMA ARE "
> FOREVER CHANGED, BOTH EMOTIONALLY
> AND PHYSICALLY.**

The impacts of trauma last long after the trauma has ended. The mind and body are connected.

---

[9] Gareth T. Jones, "Psychosocial Vulnerability and Early Life Adversity as Risk Factors for Central Sensitivity Syndromes," Current Rheumatology Reviews 12, no. 2 (June 2016): 140–53. https://doi.org/10.2174/1573397112666151231113438.

CHAPTER 10

The big "mis": Misunderstood and misdiagnosed

IBUPROFEN, INJECTIONS, AND PHYSICAL THERAPY are the go-to options for people who need treatment for pain. Over time, pain can shift—from an injury area to coming from the nervous system. This transition is easily missed. But pain from nerve sensitization doesn't respond to standard treatments, so if it is not identified, mounting frustration grows between the patient and the provider. A provider who is unfamiliar with sensitization may wrongly presume the person is drug seeking, dramatic, or trying to avoid work. The provider becomes disengaged and frustrated. Meanwhile, the patient feels heartbroken, confused, and not believed. Sensitization and its treatment are not well-known by many providers at this point, making it crucial that you choose a provider who does understand.

Here is a classic example of a back pain patient with sensitization causing the issue, where both provider and patient are unaware of the underlying cause. The patient presents with back pain. The doctor sends her to physical therapy, which does not help.

The doctor then orders an MRI. Nothing explains the severe pain level.

The doctor tries a steroid injection. The pain is not reduced.

Finally, with all these treatment options exhausted, the patient undergoes back surgery! Guess what? The pain is still there.

The patient continues to report a pain level of nine out of ten. She is fatigued every day. She can't fall asleep at night. She has brain fog at work. She files for disability because she cannot work between the pain and all the other symptoms. The confused provider doesn't see a reason for the distress level. The frustrated patient feels dismissed by the unbelieving physician. How can the provider not see her distress level? Everyone is disheartened.

This is the pattern of a patient with predominant nerve sensitization pain. The cause of the pain is no longer from the backbone or disc; it is from abnormal pain processing in the brain and nerves. Standard treatments that focus on correcting a structural problem or injury don't work because the main problem moved to the nervous system. This shift is often missed.

TREATMENT FOR BACK INJURY VS SENSITIZATION

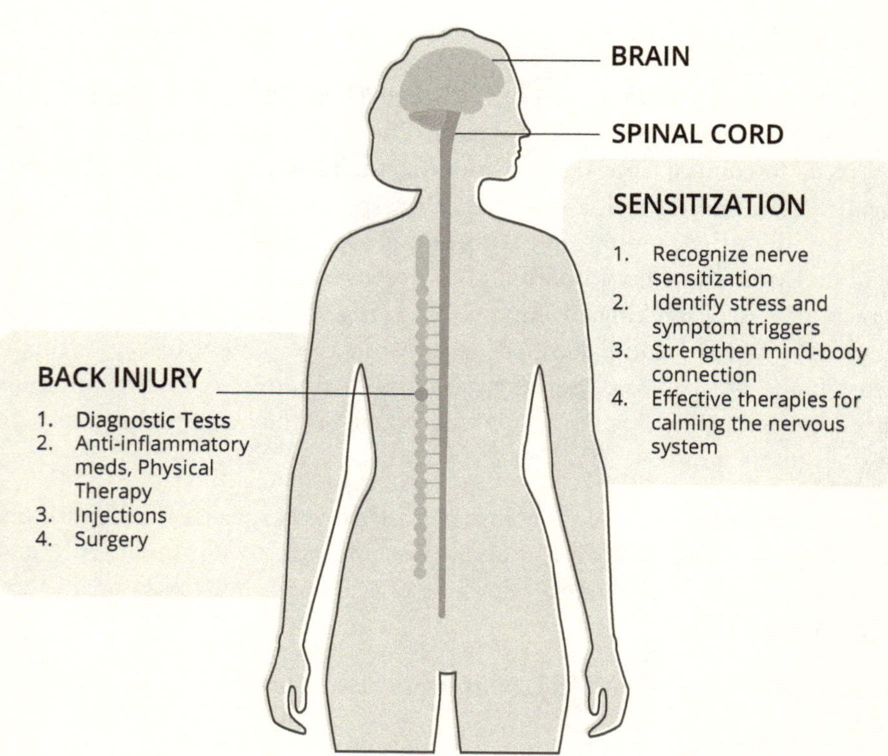

There is no surgery for disordered pain processing. In fact, since the nervous system is over-sensitive, invasive procedures can actually worsen the pain. I've told my fibromyalgia patients, "No procedures unless absolutely necessary", because the procedures don't help. And every treatment ends up hurting ten times more. The outcome from the treatments range from totally useless to horribly painful. When sensitization is driving the symptoms, the treatment approach must be different. You don't put a cast on a paralyzed arm from a stroke because the cause of the injury isn't in the arm; it's in the brain. The problem is deeper, in the nervous system. The same is true when treating a sensitization syndrome.

Studies that back up back pain

I read an enlightening study on chronic low back pain that changed the way I approach chronic pain conditions. The study examined pain sensitivity. Researchers gathered two groups of people. One group consisted of people with chronic lower back pain. The other group—the control group—had no pain.

In the study[10] researchers applied pressure to the thumbnail of each person in both groups. They asked the participants to indicate when they felt a sensation of pain of any kind, then felt moderate pain, followed by intense pain.

The point at which the participants first felt pain was significantly different between the two groups. The control group reported pain when the thumbnail pressure was at 2.7 kilograms. The chronic back pain group felt pain at only 0.7 kilograms of pressure, a fraction of the amount at which the control group felt the first inkling of pain! This pattern continued with moderate pain and severe pain.

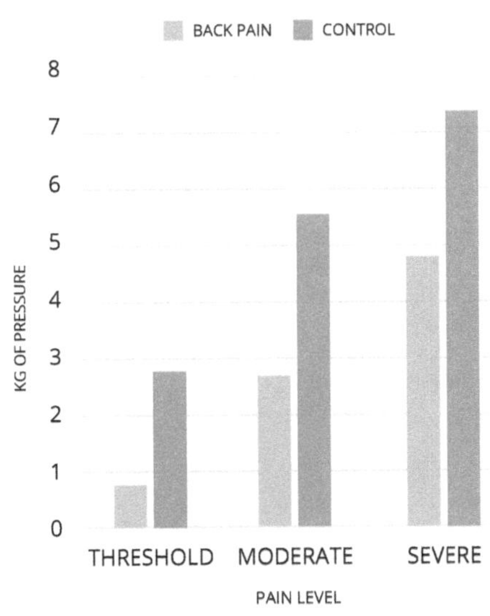

---

[10] Thorsten Giesecke et al., "Evidence of Augmented Central Pain Processing in Idiopathic Chronic Low Back Pain," Arthritis & Rheumatism 50, no. 2 (Feb 2004): 613-623.

The back pain group was more sensitive to pain, even at a site distant from their back pain. This finding supports they process pain differently.

This study also looked at what parts of the brain were activated when the participants experienced pain. Using the same pain stimulus for both groups, MRI showed that the control group activated one area of the brain, while the back pain group activated four areas. This result is visual evidence that the back pain group processed pain differently than the control group. An objective difference that providers can see, understand, and point to.

Nerve sensitization gets a new fancy name

The understanding of pain arising from abnormal sensory processing in the brain and nerves is so new that it has recently been given its own medical term, **"nociplastic pain"**.

THREE TYPES OF PAIN

In the past, pain was categorized into two types. One type, nociceptive pain, is caused by inflammation and tissue damage. It feels sharp, aching, or throbbing. The type of pain you feel when you stub your toe or sprain your ankle. Your body is telling you, "Hey, you hurt yourself."

Nociceptive Pain

The second type, neuropathic pain, arises from direct damage to nerves. The burning, tingling pain of a pinched nerve in the back, the hand numbness from carpal tunnel, or burning feet from diabetic neuropathy.

Neuropathic Pain

There is now a third type, nociplastic pain, pain arising from abnormal pain processing with no evidence of tissue damage or injury. And it has its own distinct features.[11]

Nociplastic Pain

---

[11] Mary-Ann Fitzcharles et al., "Nociplastic Pain: Towards an Understanding of Prevalent Pain Conditions," The Lancet 397, no. 10289 (May 2021): 2098–2110.

In case you nodded off during that paragraph, here's what it means....

The International Association for the Study of Pain (IASP) describes three key features of nociplastic pain as the pain arising from disordered sensory processing.[12]

1. Symptoms are chronic or long-standing. Symptoms are present for longer than three months. Disordered sensory processing develops over time. You don't strain your back and have disordered processing the next day. It evolves over months to years. In my experience, most people don't seek help until they've lived with the symptoms for a year or more. By then, their primary care provider has tried all the standard therapies or natural healing is expected to be complete.

2. Symptoms tend to spread beyond the expected area of injury. The pain area spreads or radiates to involve a greater region of the body. For example, instead of a small area of the back hurting, you feel discomfort across the back and into your legs. Someone with a pinched nerve in their neck may feel like their entire arm is numb instead of just the area supplied by the nerve.

3. Signs of increased sensitivity to painful stimuli. A lowered threshold for feeling pain develops. You feel pain more easily than those without nerve sensitization. For the injury, the pain report is much higher than expected. Or, there is pain in response to things that aren't usually painful. For instance, feeling pain with just a light touch or mild pressure on the back. Normally, light pressure on the back muscles doesn't cause discomfort outside of an injury. Nerve sensitization can result in discomfort or what appears to be exaggerated pain responses.

The lowered threshold for pain doesn't mean the person is overreacting, but rather a sign that more is happening than just a local injury. It is a clue that sensitization may be affecting symptoms. Sensitization results in the appearance of "pain out of proportion to the injury." For example, if someone breaks their leg in half and reports extreme pain, that is the expected pain level. However, if someone lightly squeezes your finger and you experience extreme pain, that response is out of proportion to the expected pain level.

Determining medical proportionality is not straightforward. Chances are, whatever pain you're feeling is new to you. A trusted and caring provider who has seen hundreds of cases should have a good radar for proportionality. You

---

[12] Jo Nijs et al., "Nociplastic Pain Criteria or Recognition of Central Sensitization? Pain Phenotyping in the Past, Present and Future," *Journal of Clinical Medicine* 10, no. 15 (July 2021): 3203. https://doi.org/10.3390/jcm10153203.

have to find a provider who is the right fit for you. Not all providers are trained in this area. If you get a blank stare or a head scratch in response to your symptoms, that provider may not be the best fit.

Mixed pain states: The injury and the sensitization

Nociplastic pain can occur by itself, such as seen in fibromyalgia, or as a mixed pain state where there is an injury plus sensitization causing pain signals, as with chronic low back pain. A mixed pain state happens when multiple sources of pain develop; pain coming from an injured area, like the back, and pain from disordered sensory processing. In this way, it is like treating two disorders. The difficulty is the two overlap into one set of symptoms.

MIXED PAIN STATES

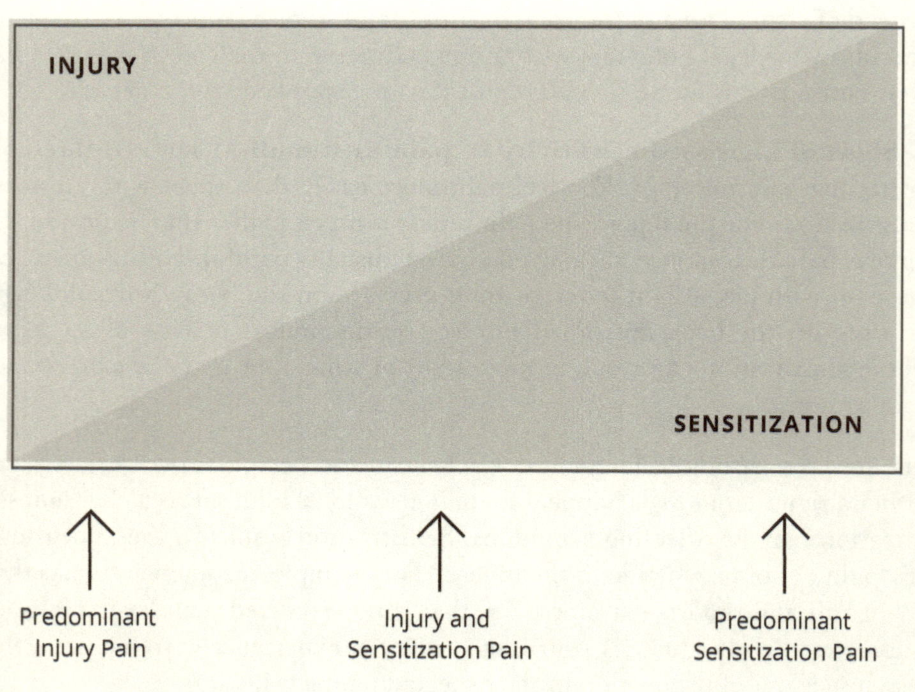

A common example is chronic back pain. Discomfort can arise from two different sources:

1. The injury area, a herniated back disc; and/or

2. Amplified pain from nerve sensitization.

Sensitization increases the pain signal that is already present. Sensitization can even perpetuate the pain after the injury signals are gone!

Spectrum of sensitization

You can experience back pain from an injury with no sensitization; this situation will respond well to standard treatments.

You can have chronic back pain with some sensitization; in this case, there will be a partial response to standard treatments.

But if you have back pain with predominant sensitization—like Melissa's case where most of the symptoms stemmed from sensitization—there is minimal response to standard treatments.

Standard treatments don't work when the pain is predominantly from sensitization because the dysfunction has shifted to the nervous system. The more that sensitization is driving the symptoms, the less responsive they are to standard treatments.

Same pain, different problems

Linda and Nicole both had lower back pain. They both showed sciatic-like symptoms, with pain shooting down the leg. Each woman underwent the same treatments, but had different responses.

Herniated disc. Linda's back pain came from a herniated disc that was irritating a nerve. She had burning pain running down the back of her leg for a few days. She had no indicators of sensitization (disordered pain processing). For treatment, Linda received a steroid injection. She had significant improvement. Her pain level went from ten to four. She took nerve pain medication (gabapentin) for about six months. By nine months, Linda no longer had symptoms and weaned off the medication. Linda's clinical picture is consistent with pain from a local injury, a disc herniation, without sensitization. Her symptoms resolved as the injury healed.

Nerve sensitization. Nicole's back and leg pain had been present for a year. She, too, had burning pain radiating down the back of her leg. She had many indicators of sensitization. The pain spread far beyond the low back and nerve. Her entire low back, back of her thighs, and leg hurt. Nicole underwent a steroid injection but it did not help. She experienced other symptoms too, like difficulty sleeping at night and daily fatigue. She missed a lot of work because of the pain. Some days, Nicole just couldn't function. Nicole's clinical picture fits with pain from nerve sensitization.

Two people with similar symptoms, but different responses to treatment. Their responses differed because the source of their pain differed. Linda had a structural cause, a herniated disc. It caused swelling. The pain fibers signaled. The steroid reduced the swelling, which reduced the pain signal firing. The nerve calmed down over time. The body healed the structural issue over the next six months.

Nicole, however, had disordered pain processing from nerve sensitization. There was no swelling irritating the nerve. Instead, Nicole's disordered pain processing kept telling her brain she was hurt. Although an injury may have started the pain, it was no longer a predominant factor. The non-pain symptoms of difficulty sleeping and daily fatigue were clues that nerve sensitization was present. Nerve sensitization maintained the pain even after the injury healed.

Since the source of Linda and Nicole's pain is different, their treatments are different. Linda did well with standard treatments. Nicole requires treatment for nerve sensitization.

You need to be aware of sensitization to prevent undergoing procedures that won't help. Procedures not only fail to help with nerve sensitization, but may worsen the pain. If nerves are over-sensitive and over-reactive, the last thing you want to do is take a scalpel to the area and make more pain inputs that will be amplified and sent to the brain! Sadly, I have seen many examples of this problem in my practice. Patients were unaware and so desperate for relief that they followed every recommendation. I don't want this to happen to you! Beware of a surgeon with rose-colored Versace glasses.

BOTTOM LINE

Nerve sensitization treatment requires an approach that targets disordered sensory processing. I will go more in-depth in the following chapters but, for now, you should know that the treatment is much broader, because multiple areas are involved—the source of the injury and the dysfunction in the nerves. At the same time, treatment is more targeted due to each individual's unique clinical needs. You can't rely on algorithms here; they don't consider the ways one person's needs, triggers, and physiology differ from another's. One person may require medications that calm the over-responsive nerves to help "reset" them. Another person may need stress reduction and training on the mind-body or "stress-body" connection. For most, incorporating regular exercise, good nutrition, and adequate sleep are helpful.

CHAPTER 11

Is everything really ok? Learn the symptoms

LET ME KEEP HAMMERING ON this point. Standard treatments that focus on correcting a structural problem or injury do not work if the problem is sensitization. So how can you assess if it is an issue? Well, certain patterns suggest sensitization is a factor.

The signs of sensitization

- symptoms persist long past the expected healing time

- symptoms spread beyond the boundary of the injury area

- marked increase in sensitivity to painful stimuli

- non-pain symptoms that cause system-wide symptoms like severe fatigue, disrupted sleep, and brain fog

Beyond looking for the pattern, you can use a clinical tool, a symptom evaluator, for a more objective assessment. The clinical tool is called the central sensitization inventory (CSI).[13]

The CSI addresses common sensitization symptoms, non-pain symptoms, and associated mental health conditions. The tool consists of 25 statements. About half of them refer to symptoms of sensitization syndromes, such as headaches

---

[13] Tom G. Mayer et al., "The Development and Psychometric Validation of the Central Sensitization Inventory," Pain Practice 12, no. 4 (September 2011): 276–85. https://doi.org/10.1111/j.1533-2500.2011.00493.x.

and stiff, achy muscles. The other questions are used to gather information about the non-pain symptoms, such as sleep issues and fatigue.

For example, the first statement says, *I feel tired and unrefreshed when I wake from sleeping.*

Another states, *I get tired very easily when I am physically active.*

The measure also considers associated factors, including stress, mental health, and prior trauma. The CSI looks at whether stress makes physical symptoms worse. It asks about anxiety attacks, feeling sad, and about any trauma suffered as a child. All are additional aspects in the development or worsening of sensitization syndromes.

The CSI score is calculated by assigning scores of zero, one, two, three, or four to the response categories ranging from "never" to "always." After answering the questions, your total score is calculated within a range from zero to one hundred, with higher scores suggesting more sensitization. A score of forty or higher is indicative of significant symptoms from sensitization.

The purpose of the CSI tool is to develop awareness of potential sensitization symptoms. The measure is not meant as a self-diagnostic tool since diagnosis requires consideration of other factors not included in it.

The inventory is a useful list of all the different symptoms that sensitization of the nervous system can cause. I encourage you to study this tool. You can repeat it every few weeks to monitor symptoms or response to therapy.

NOTE: Diagnosis of sensitization syndrome should be done by a licensed medical provider. While the CSI is helpful to get started, you could have an undiagnosed medical condition along with nerve sensitization. The tool doesn't evaluate for the possibility of overlapping medical conditions that cause the same symptoms. For example, low thyroid can cause the symptoms listed here, such as fatigue, sadness, and digestive changes. And, of course, you can have both at once. Due to the complicated nature of the diagnosis, be sure to seek a qualified provider for an evaluation.

CENTRAL SENSITIZATION INVENTORY

Please circle the best response to the right of each statement.

1	I feel tired and unrefreshed when I wake from sleeping.	Never	Rarely	Sometimes	Often	Always
2	My muscles feel stiff and achy.	Never	Rarely	Sometimes	Often	Always
3	I have anxiety attacks.	Never	Rarely	Sometimes	Often	Always
4	I grind or clench my teeth.	Never	Rarely	Sometimes	Often	Always
5	I have problems with diarrhea and/or constipation.	Never	Rarely	Sometimes	Often	Always
6	I need help in performing my daily activities.	Never	Rarely	Sometimes	Often	Always
7	I am sensitive to bright lights.	Never	Rarely	Sometimes	Often	Always
8	I get tired very easily when I am physically active.	Never	Rarely	Sometimes	Often	Always
9	I feel pain all over my body.	Never	Rarely	Sometimes	Often	Always
10	I have headaches.	Never	Rarely	Sometimes	Often	Always
11	I feel discomfort in my bladder and/or burning when I urinate.	Never	Rarely	Sometimes	Often	Always
12	I do not sleep well.	Never	Rarely	Sometimes	Often	Always
13	I have difficulty concentrating.	Never	Rarely	Sometimes	Often	Always
14	I have skin problems such as dryness, itchiness, or rashes.	Never	Rarely	Sometimes	Often	Always
15	Stress makes my physical symptoms get worse.	Never	Rarely	Sometimes	Often	Always
16	I feel sad or depressed.	Never	Rarely	Sometimes	Often	Always
17	I have low energy.	Never	Rarely	Sometimes	Often	Always
18	I have muscle tension in my neck and shoulders.	Never	Rarely	Sometimes	Often	Always
19	I have pain in my jaw.	Never	Rarely	Sometimes	Often	Always
20	Certain smells, such as perfumes, make me feel dizzy and nauseated.	Never	Rarely	Sometimes	Often	Always
21	I have to urinate frequently.	Never	Rarely	Sometimes	Often	Always
22	My legs feel uncomfortable and restless when I am trying to go to sleep at night.	Never	Rarely	Sometimes	Often	Always
23	I have difficulty remembering things.	Never	Rarely	Sometimes	Often	Always
24	I suffered trauma as a child.	Never	Rarely	Sometimes	Often	Always
25	I have pain in my pelvic area.	Never	Rarely	Sometimes	Often	Always
					Total=	

Developed at **PRIDE**. The CSI questionnaire is available for free download at pridedallas.com

BOTTOM LINE

The central sensitization inventory lists potential sensitization symptoms. As basic as it sounds, understanding sensitization and its contribution to symptoms is an important step. Melissa told me that gaining this awareness was the most helpful tool for managing her chronic low back pain. She finally understood why she was experiencing pain. This knowledge lowered Melissa's fear and anxiety. She gained the peace of mind she needed to work through the pain because she was confident that nothing catastrophic or life-threatening was happening. This comfort also lowered her stress response.

Understanding what is happening and why returns a sense of control and an improved ability to manage the symptoms.

Knowing you are going to be ok and not in danger is a big relief. The emotional centers of the brain that latch onto fear and turn up the pain volume won't be triggered as often when you have peace of mind. You can maintain control and self-manage better.

CHAPTER 12

SunRISE Process: Start your path to healing

HEALING STARTS WITH BECOMING AWARE of sensitization and stress effects on your body, the mind-body connection. As we saw in Melissa's case, when sensitization is present, the treatment approach is different. The direction shifts away from targeting a local injury and broadens to addressing the nervous system.

To manage symptoms from sensitization or stress, you must first be aware it is a factor. It is hard to fix a problem when you don't know it exists.

When I worked in the stroke recovery unit, we saw a common feature with "left" brain strokes versus "right" brain strokes.

With a left brain stroke, the patient tends to have insight into their deficits from the stroke. They are aware they can't swallow or walk safely. Because of this awareness, they tend to be more melancholy. They also tend to have more potential to improve with rehab because they know what they need to work on. Because of their awareness, even with impaired swallowing from their stroke, they are careful when they eat and there are few problems with choking.

Meanwhile, those with a right brain stroke have much less insight into their deficits. They choke more on food and fall more when trying to walk, even with milder deficits. Without awareness of a deficit, it is hard to compensate for it. Safety is a constant challenge since they don't realize their balance is off, so they stand impulsively and fall repeatedly. The right brain strokes have a harder time in rehab since they have limited awareness of what they need to work on.

RISE and shine

Before you can manage the symptoms of sensitization and the impact of stress, you have to build awareness of how they present in you. The SunRISE process helps you recognize sensitization in yourself, identify stress and the physical symptoms it causes (stress-body connection), and strengthens this connection with mindfulness practice—along with exploring effective therapies to calm over-vigilant nerves and decrease the pain level.

SunRISE PROCESS

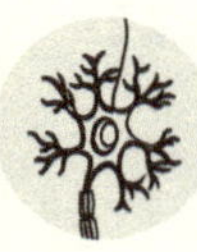 **R**ecognize nerve sensitization

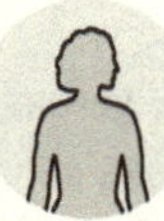 **I**dentify stress + make the stress-body connection

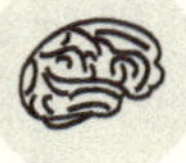 **S**trengthen connection with mindfulness practice

 **E**ffective therapies to calm the nervous system

Let's look at each step—what it is, why it matters, and how to get there.

1. Recognize nerve sensitization

Chronic lower back pain—like Melissa's—is a common sensitization syndrome. In her case, sensitization was the predominant driver of her symptoms and included the non-pain symptoms of fatigue and brain fog. When Melissa's back pain flared, her fatigue levels and brain fog also worsened. Her functional level decreased for days, and she needed time to rest and recover. With improved awareness, Melissa now knows she is ok. She sees these symptoms as signals that she overdid it. Her body screams at her in a more "intense" way to lower demands because of the sensitization. She must prioritize her health.

> UNDERSTAND THE BODY'S MESSAGE.
> THEN, LISTEN TO IT WITHOUT SHAME
> OR JUDGMENT.

When it comes to building awareness of symptoms from sensitization, a helpful starting point is the central sensitization inventory (CSI), which I've discussed previously. The CSI helps build awareness of sensitization symptoms and the factors that worsen it. The inventory reviews the pain symptoms and non-pain symptoms, as well as related factors like stress, mental health, and trauma. If you find yourself nodding "yes" as you scroll through the list, it is a sign that sensitization may be contributing.

Understanding recalibrates the "freak-out" meter.

As Melissa discovered, understanding that sensitization is present and contributing to symptoms made a difference. She received confirmation that the pain wasn't something she imagined or exaggerated. Melissa found it reassuring that a symptom flare-up was related to sensitization rather than a new or worsening injury. When you know you are going to be "ok", you're in a better mindset to manage your symptoms.

With time, you see a pattern to your symptoms, which, in turn, builds confidence that you can work through it. A greater sense of control and less fear emerges. This, in and of itself, reduces suffering. Once you understand your pattern, management becomes easier. You can confidently resume activities you enjoy. And know to avoid some others! This is the first glimmer of light. The beginning of your own sunbreak.

2. Identify stress and make the stress-body connection

Bryan's experience with chronic headaches represents another common sensitization syndrome. Within a CSS, sensitization can increase symptoms anywhere from a mild to a severe amount; it occurs across a spectrum. A CSI score greater than 40 suggests significant sensitization symptoms are present. Melissa's CSI score was 59. Sensitization was a significant contributor to her pain level. By contrast, Bryan's main issue was that high stress levels triggered headaches. His CSI score was 17; he had minimal sensitization affecting his pain level.

Sensitization syndromes have predictable triggers that worsen symptoms. High stress is a frequent one. Work stress is a big one, especially when the demands are high and the control of the situation is low. For example, you're working against continuous tight deadlines or high stakes with no control over work volume or resources. Think about those situations when perfection is required but the time or resources for it are not available. For Bryan, perfection was a must; each project had to be perfect and completed on a tight timeline. But, the work volume overwhelmed his company's resources. The work demands were unrealistic and unsustainable.

Bryan needed to grasp the stress-body connection. When his headaches flared, he had to reduce work demands to bring his headaches under control. When he kept his stress levels manageable, he kept his headaches manageable. Understanding the stress-body connection was key to managing his CSS.

To build your stress-body connection, start by exploring how stress presents physically in you. Here is a hint: Stress likes to exploit our weak links. Bad back? Feel it there. Bad shoulder? The pain hits there. Sensitive stomach? That's where it goes. Prone to headaches? You'll probably feel the stress in your head. Similar to how stress expressed itself in the people we have met, Melissa's back hurt, Bryan had piercing eye pain, and Olivia had miserable bladder pain.

Starting an **Awareness Journal** helps you see how your stress shows physically. It helps build the stress-body connection. When symptoms flare, write down what you are feeling physically and emotionally. Write down where you feel the symptoms, what you are doing, and how you are feeling. Write the emotions—like sad, frustrated, disappointed, worried, confused, or angry. Get in the habit of labeling the emotions you are feeling. And, let yourself feel them. Over time, this process reveals patterns and symptom triggers.

Awareness Journal

Date: _______________________

Symptom Location: Headache

My mood today: 😁 🙂 😐 😒 🙁 😫

Symptom Intensity: ◯ ◯ ◯ ◯ ⊗ ◯ ◯ ◯ ◯ ◯
          1 2 3 4 5 6 7 8 9 10

What I was doing when my symptoms started:
I was working on travel arrangements for my in-laws,
having technical issues with my computer.

How I felt when my symptoms started:
Frustrated by computer, irritable.

Anything unique about the day or coming up in the next week:
In-laws are coming to visit.

MARK IF YOU FEEL ANY PAIN

FRONT   BACK

After keeping an Awareness Journal for two weeks, check for patterns. Are there certain activities that consistently result in increased symptoms? Do certain emotions consistently intensify symptoms?

For example, let's say a mom's four-year-old son with ADHD loses control every time she takes him to the doctor's office. Each time, they have to wait for 30 minutes before they are seen. During these 30 minutes, her son runs all over the clinic. He has no self-regulation or control of himself. If she takes him outside, he dashes into traffic. Once mom gets him in the exam room, he tears the room apart. She notices that every time they have a doctor's appointment, she gets a headache. There is a clear pattern that taking her son to the doctor's office gives her a headache due to how difficult it is. Now that she has made the connection, she can take action to reduce this trigger and the headaches. She changes to the first appointment of the day to eliminate the wait and brings an engaging toy for him to play with. The appointments are shorter and easier to get through. Her headaches improve. This is how an Awareness Journal can help show the stress-body connection.

The Awareness Journal shows patterns that are easily overlooked otherwise. In the beginning, you may not realize your triggers or the degree of stress you're bearing. Your awareness may start slowly, but it will grow with time. With each journal entry, the picture becomes clearer. It is a process that shows itself with consistent practice.

Another clinical tool that helps make the stress-body connection is the **Perceived Stress Scale (PSS)**. The level of stress we are under is hard to see in ourselves, especially when it builds slowly over time. What was supposed to be one hard month becomes every single day over years. We just soak it up, fooling ourselves into believing, "I've got this."

The PSS provides a more objective perspective of your stress level. The scale measures your perceived stress level. This is an important point since what we perceive as stressful is what activates the body's stress response. To be clear, it is not what we think should be stressful, but what our body actually perceives as stressful. These may be two different things!

For instance, I don't think my son's asthma attacks should be stressful because I know if the attack becomes severe, I can give him oral steroids and it will help. In 30 minutes, his breathing will stabilize. Yet, during that 30-minute time period when his eyes are welling with tears, he is clutching his throat, and struggling to move air, my stress response launches into overdrive! What I think should be stressful and what my body finds stressful don't agree.

The Perceived Stress Scale consists of ten questions that assess how unpredictable, uncontrollable, and overloaded we feel in life. It assesses stress levels over the past month. I'm not able to reprint the questionnaire here due to copyright, but it is available with an internet search. Sample questions include:

- In the last month, how often have you felt that you were unable to control the important things in your life?

- In the last month, how often have you felt confident about your ability to handle your personal problems?

- In the last month, how often have you felt you were on top of things?

Responses are scored on a continuum from 0 to 4, from "never" to "very often". Your total score ranges from zero to 40 with higher scores indicating higher perceived stress. Scores ranging from zero to 13 are considered low stress, 14 to 26 moderate stress, and 27 to 40 high stress.

A higher score, such as one that falls in the moderate or high range, may provide awareness to make a needed change. When I used this tool myself, I found I was more stressed than I realized. Before using the PSS, I estimated I was mildly stressed; however, my score placed me as moderately stressed. Once this was brought to my attention, I realized that I struggled more than I admitted, more than I thought I should be. My results prompted me to figure out a few more resources for my son. The measure helped me identify my actual stress level without allowing my personal judgment to cloud reality. Going forward, I feel more in tune with my actual stress level.

3. Strengthen the mind-body connection with mindfulness

Mindfulness refers to living in the present moment as opposed to being lost in thought. For example, standing in the kitchen first thing in the morning and feeling the sunshine on your skin rather than thinking about your work meeting with your difficult colleague, Karen. Meditation and mindful exercise (e.g. yoga) are other ways to practice mindfulness. The practice elevates awareness of yourself, your body, and the connection between them.

Mindfulness practice changes how your brain processes information. You are able to separate from your thoughts and emotions, allowing the real you to emerge. You are in control of your thoughts and emotions, rather than them controlling you. You are able to enjoy the life you are living now, in the present moment, rather than existing in the worries of your mind.

4. Effective therapies to calm the nervous system

If sensitization pain is filling your day with suffering, there are medication and non-medication therapies that help calm over-reactive nerves and lower the pain level—medications that are specific to nerve and sensitization pain. Acupuncture has also shown benefits. In addition, complementary treatments with physical therapy, chiropractic care, and massage therapy have a role, depending on the type of CSS.

In the next sections, I will go into more detail about key stress management tips, then dive into how to strengthen the mind-body connection (S) and effective medical therapies (E).

—————————————————— BOTTOM LINE ——————————————————

Healing starts with becoming aware of sensitization and stress effects on your body. The SunRISE process guides you through how to recognize nerve sensitization, identify stressors and make the stress-body connection. Tracking your CSI score, keeping an Awareness Journal, and following your PSS score all help build this connection. Mindfulness practice strengthens the stress-body connection.

CHAPTER 13

Small things make a big difference: Stress management strategies

"Psychological factors can modulate the stress response. Perceive yourself in a given situation to have expressive outlets, control, and predictive information, for example, and you are less likely to have a stress response."

—Robert Sapolsky

WE'VE REVIEWED SOME WAYS TO assess stress levels, so let's touch on some basic stress management techniques. But first, I need to give two important caveats.

One, the first step requires evaluating whether you can realistically manage the stress or a greater change is needed. Stress management strategies are useful, but no amount of meditation or mindfulness will resolve unrealistic demands.

Two, these stress management techniques are meant to deal with the stress culture of Western lifestyle. The hustle culture, lean in, do-it-all, mind-over-matter, until-you're-disabled culture. The stress management strategies here are not meant for those in disastrous situations. They do not apply to the family struggling to feed their kids, procure housing, or receive basic medical care. They don't apply to those suffering abuse. They don't apply to those fleeing war-torn countries. These strategies are intended to help with Western hustle culture.

> **"** STRESS MANAGEMENT STRATEGIES ARE
> USEFUL, BUT NO AMOUNT OF MEDITATION
> OR MINDFULNESS WILL RESOLVE
> UNREALISTIC DEMANDS. **"**

Manage your stress

In his book on stress, *Why Zebras Don't Get Ulcers,* Sapolsky presents key strategies to help manage, manageable stress.

Strategy 1: Social support—We need each other.

If the COVID pandemic taught me anything, it was the importance of meaningful social connections. Sapolsky discusses the importance of the right social support—support from people who are actually helpful. A supportive partner, the right network of friends, and the right community. As opposed to those who may make you feel judged or weak. Or a group where you just don't feel you belong.

Strategy 2: Regular exercise—Any movement you enjoy works!

Whether walking, bunny hops, or burpees, the concept of "anything is better than nothing" applies here. Exercise is a natural anti-stressor. It enhances mood and blunts the stress response. A daily 20-minute or one-mile walk does wonders for your physical and mental health.

I encourage the practice of mindful exercise, such as yoga. Yoga combines movement, breath work, and the practice of presence—being in the moment, and not letting your attention stray. Breath work calms the stress response. Meanwhile, the postures strengthen the core muscles in the stomach and back and restore healthy joint motion. Your thoughts are put on pause and your mind is decluttered. When your mind comes back online, it is more clear, detached, and at peace.

Mindful exercise and yoga have a variety of different forms. Different styles focus more on the elements of movement, meditation, or breathwork. Chances are, you can find a practice that works for you. For example, vinyasa yoga is a more athletic style where you flow from pose to pose; it feels like a more traditional workout. Yin yoga is slower paced. Each pose is held for one to two minutes and the focus is on a deep stretch. Yoga as a base for workouts has expanded into popular fusion workouts that combine the best of yoga with the benefits of other modalities. For example, adding weights and resistance bands to the workouts.

This type of exercise is particularly good for strengthening your mind-body connection, knowing when the body is signaling for help. It is a great option for those recovering from a stress-related disorder, if you enjoy it.

Strategy 3: Outlets—Schedule them.

Stress-relieving outlets are activities that you enjoy, that put you in a flow state—the psychology term for when you are fully immersed in an activity. Activities so enjoyable you lose all sense of time and are truly in the moment. Activities where you can detach from the day's stress. You are not thinking about what happened at the meeting earlier that day and you are not thinking about the work project due next week. You are engrossed in the moment.

Stress-relieving outlets may include a favorite hobby or passion project. Exercise or art. Music or a nature walk. Listening to Dr. Sapolsky YouTube videos about physiology. Whatever you enjoy.

Schedule your stress-relieving outlets into the week, prioritize it!

Strategy 4: Journaling—Get it out of your head.

Journaling is a great way to unburden the mind and relieve stress.

Thought journaling is writing down your thoughts, your feelings, and your frustrations. This simple act allows you to process them at a deeper level. Take 20 minutes and write exactly what is on your mind at that moment and how you feel about it. Go deep. Write down your deepest emotions and painful conflicts. Any thoughts circling on repeat in your mind, write them down. You can shred it and throw it in the garbage later. Let go and explore your thoughts, knowing no one will ever see it. Journal each day or once a week, whichever helps you process. It is a simple, effective way to work through emotions and move past conflicts.

With gratitude journaling, you write what you are grateful for. In doing so, you reset your mind on a positive path. Focusing on gratitude refreshes positive thoughts and brings about positive emotions. This exercise is a wonderful way to quickly boost your mood.

Try it now. Think of three things you are grateful for. It can be as simple as having a great cup of coffee in the morning or a pleasant conversation with a stranger. Maybe you're grateful that your child is happy and thriving.

Read out loud what you are grateful for. Notice how your mind adjusts. Gratitude journaling redirects the subconscious on a positive path, then the conscious mind follows.

Strategy 5: Mindfulness practice—Live your actual life.

Mindfulness practice can take various forms, from focusing on living in the moment during your day to a meditation practice to mindful exercise (e.g., yoga). I am still a novice, yet I'm amazed at how it has calmed my mind and lightened my heart. The practice of mindfulness has clarified what's truly important and highlighted the petty in a way I could not appreciate before. With this distinction, I can filter out the noise and focus on what matters. The concepts reviewed in Eckhart Tolle's book, Stillness Speaks, gave me my start. Living in the now, calming non-productive thoughts, and quieting the ego were transformative.

From mindfulness, I branched into mindful forms of exercise. I tried several yoga styles but vinyasa flow was my favorite. I love efficiency, so getting in my mindfulness practice and exercise at once is a satisfying activity.

As the benefits from daily mindfulness and mindful exercise grew, I started working on a meditation practice. Similar to mindful exercise, meditation has many different forms. Even 15 minutes a day of meditation enables you to detach and distance yourself from the mind's overbearing emotions or negative thought streams. Meditation connects you with your inner essence, the real you. The process helps separate you from the mind-made you, crafted from labeling, judgments, and distorted perceptions.

Over the years, I have gained control over where my mind goes. I am less reactive. I handle stressful situations better. I can better manage my thoughts and emotions. They are no longer controlling me.

Mind-body work—such as the practice of mindfulness, meditation, and mindful exercise—reduces the stress response. Mindfulness practice reverses stress physiology to normal physiology, a real power tool for coping with and managing stress.

Strategy 6: Sleep—It helps...a lot.

Everything feels worse without sleep. Sleep deprivation increases pain levels, worsens fatigue, and makes it harder to cope with stress. The quality of sleep is just as important as the amount of sleep. Here are tips to improve sleep.

- Clear your mind. A few ideas to calm your mind before bed include: writing a to-do list of items on your mind, journaling about your day, or meditating.

- Minimize late-day caffeine. Find your absolute caffeine cut-off point during the day. The latest time of the day you can consume caffeine without it interfering with falling asleep. For some, it's noon; for others, it's 4pm. If you need a slight pick me up later in the day, opt for ginger tea instead. Ginger tea provides a boost in energy and focus.

- Filter the screens. Although it's ideal not to look at screens a couple of hours before bed, if you do, try a blue light filter, such as blue light glasses. Light—and notably blue light—interferes with the release of melatonin, the bedtime hormone that helps you fall asleep.

- Keep it cool. You get the best sleep in a cool room, target between 65 to70 degrees Fahrenheit.

- Keep a consistent sleep schedule. Go to sleep and wake up around the same time every day.

- Regular exercise. Get the wiggles out before bedtime. Try 20 to 30 minutes of exercise each day, most days of the week. Brisk walking counts!

If you consistently have trouble falling asleep at night, waking up multiple times per night, or waking up unrefreshed, talk with your provider to make sure there is not an underlying medical issue to consider, such as sleep apnea.

BOTTOM LINE

When it comes to stress management, the first step is determining if your stress is manageable or requires a greater change. By greater change, I mean adjustments to how your life looks and how you function each day, such as your job, where you live, etc. Once you've determined your stress is manageable, the following stress management tips may help:

- Seek social support from the right people, where you feel you belong.

- Exercise regularly, any movement works.

- Schedule activities each week that you enjoy.

- Write down your thoughts, including gratitude, in a journal.

- Practice mindfulness—from enjoying the moment to mindful exercise to meditation; ten minutes a day is all it takes to see the benefits.

- Aim for quality sleep, which makes coping with stress easier.

CHAPTER 14

How mindfulness practice shapes brain health

MINDFULNESS IS MORE THAN JUST a stress management technique. The practice of mindfulness changes neurocircuitry, so you think and react in a healthier, more adaptive way...an evolution over time producing a calm, detached, responsive awareness. It brings you closer to your authentic self, your inner essence, the real you.

In its simplest form, mindfulness refers to living in the present moment, aware and receptive to what's happening around you. This is the starting point for the practice of mindfulness. In Western culture, we find ourselves immersed in thoughts about past events or future endeavors. Our mind wanders off and we miss the actual now.

Looking back, I missed most of my twenties. I was entirely focused on the future, the next medical school exam, then the next medical rotation, then residency, then post-residency training. Always focused on the next hurdle. There was no balance, no appreciation for where I was in the moment. There was no present consciousness. I was the proverbial rat running a race, with little awareness. When I completed medical training in my early thirties, I thought I should try living my actual life, instead of being lost in thoughts about the future of it. That was the gentle start to my practice of mindfulness.

Let me be honest, that was the gentle start following a scandalous divorce that shook the ground beneath my feet. I married an emergency room doctor. He enjoyed the flattery of a few to a dozen nurses. He enjoyed their company, intimately. 'Til nurse do us part.

I fell right out of the rat race and woke up to more than the failure of my marriage. As my husband prepared to leave that night, he condescendingly asked me how I could not have noticed his affairs. He handed me his phone to show me the texts from one of his girlfriends. Undaunted, he looked at me one last time as he walked out the door and said, "There are a lot of people who want to spend time with me." In retrospect, the infidelity was merely a symptom of a union not meant to be. He did me a favor that night by jolting me awake to my mistake, and my life.

Mindfulness practice types

The practice of mindfulness starts and looks in many different ways. For me, it started with intentionally being aware a few hours each day. A few hours where I did not think about the next day or the next task and did not analyze the previous day's events. I remained in the present moment. I inserted a pause into the constant thought stream of all the patient care activities from the day. It also included being present and listening to patients, as opposed to focusing on collecting their interim clinical data, adjusting the plan, and moving on to the next, barely making eye contact. Rather, being present with them, being present with their struggle, being present for their needs.

You can start your own mindfulness practice by spending some time each day focusing on staying in the moment. Soaking in and being aware of the environment around you. Sitting down for your morning coffee, tea, or breakfast, pay attention to the flavor. Don't let your mind wander off to thoughts about work. Look outside, pay attention to the birds sitting on the lawn. Don't think about your to-do list. Walk outside, pay attention to the trees, how green they are and how they move with the wind.

Another option to practice mindfulness is to start a meditation program. Here is the simple and effective meditation technique I use. At a calm moment of my day, often late at night, I go to a tranquil room in my house. Others may enjoy an outside location. I set a timer for fifteen minutes so I don't think or worry about time. As I sit in a comfortable position, I focus on my breath, paying attention to breathing in and out. I don't think or follow any thought streams that pop up. If a thought does pop up, I do not follow it; I refocus on my breath. I have continual intrusive thoughts so I say "in" as I breathe in and say "out" as I breathe out; this helps me pause my thoughts. When I am focusing on my breath, an intrusive thought cannot sneak in. This allows me to clear my mind. It's a mindful blockade.

During meditation, think of your thoughts as clouds. You are monitoring them, watching them, and letting them pass. Focus on blue skies. If the sky fills with clouds, refocus on your breath, refocus on the blue sky. Learning to control your thoughts is one of the skills meditation brings. It takes effort and practice to regulate your thoughts. Start with just five minutes a day and work up to ten to twenty minutes a day. Find what works for you.

Mindfulness meditation with a breath focus is helpful for me because it is simple and pauses my thought stream. My mind is naturally wired to be on the more neurotic end of things; I worry, so meditation provides a much-needed counterbalance. Over months and years, I have felt my brain evolve to a healthier way of responding to the environment. I am naturally more mindful during the day with less effort. The benefits grew from a few hours of intentional awareness each day and ten minutes of meditation a few times per week.

MEDITATION IS THE CLOSEST TOOL TO A RESET BUTTON FOR YOUR BRAIN.

Meditation is the closest tool to a reset button for your brain, providing a fresh perspective without the residue of the previous day's events blurring the view. Mindfulness meditation and transcendental meditation are common forms. Find the style that suits you.

Mindful exercise combines the mind-calming effects of meditation with physical movement. It is the ultimate mind-body exercise as you are simultaneously working on emotional health and physical health.

Yoga is a form of mindful exercise consisting of a series of body poses that you move through slowly or quickly depending on the style. Tai chi is another popular type. An alternative to yoga involving a series of movements done in a slow way without pauses. Tai chi is described as "meditation in motion"—a continuous flow of body movement.

With so many different varieties of mindful exercise—from slower to faster paced and low to high intensity—you can find the style that meets your needs. Or make up a style that is perfect for you!

Getting chill

Mindfulness is the practice of cultivating awareness of your present experience—in the moment—of the life you are living right now. Experiencing a moment without having an opinion or judgment about it. Just accepting it as it is. Not resisting it. Mindfulness promotes awareness and equanimity. Equanimity is mental calmness and composure even in a difficult situation—to be "chill".

Present-day research supports the effectiveness of mindfulness practice and its benefits. The practice improves self-regulation, including your ability to control your attention, thoughts, and emotions.[14] Specifically, what we pay attention to, our emotional response, and what we think about. This not only sounds good but feels good…healthier. The mind—and your world—feels calmer, lighter, and more controlled.

Emotions influence our perception of events, our thinking, and our behavior. Emotional regulation is the ability to be aware of your emotions and respond to them in a healthy way. To have a controlled response rather than an emotionally charged, regrettable, reactive response. Mindfulness improves the ability to deal effectively with challenges.

For example, mindfulness enables you to stay detached and objective in a conflict and not let emotions derail a productive discussion. If a coworker is emotionally distressed and complaining to you, you don't take it personally, getting agitated and defensive in response. Instead, you accept that the coworker is frustrated, and, without judgment, consider the best response. Maybe you determine the person just needs to vent and you listen. Maybe you determine they are bringing up an important problem. By accepting and not judging the moment, you are able to respond productively. You are in a more peaceful, observational state where you can objectively appraise a situation before responding. Mindfulness enables this ability—acceptance and non-judgment of experiences with a controlled response.

" MINDFULNESS IS AKIN TO BRAIN STRENGTH " TRAINING.

Mindfulness is akin to brain strength training, improving the ability to control your thoughts and emotions, so they don't control you. Before I started my practice, the mindfulness definition "enables acceptance and non-judgment of experiences" didn't make sense to me. What does that even mean? Over the past ten years with my practice, I now understand what it means because I can do it. Well, I can do it about half of the time! You have to have faith in the first few months that change is coming because it is hard to understand before you achieve it, but you will!

---

[14] Zev Schuman-Olivier et al., "Mindfulness and Behavior Change," Harvard Review of Psychiatry 28, no. 6 (November/December 2020): 371–394. https://doi.org/10.1097/hrp.0000000000000277.

Mindfulness and perspective shifting

Mindfulness fosters the ability to shift perspectives. Known as "cognitive reappraisal", it is a healthy strategy to cope with negative emotions. This method involves taking a different perspective on a situation. Shift to a more neutral standpoint that reduces your negative emotions. You shift from a biased, negative perspective to a more neutral one. For example, let's say your back pain is flaring. Instead of thinking, "My back pain is destroying my life; I can't do anything," you switch to a more neutral statement: "My back pain is flaring today. I am going to need to rest. It is usually better in two days." The second statement is more neutral, healthier, and closer to reality. You appraise what you're feeling from a positive mindset. Still true, you're not deluding yourself, but looking at it from a neutral standpoint.

Perspective shifting requires effort when first starting, but with time your mind will start to naturally shift. Get started by writing down on the left hand side of a piece of paper three negative thoughts you have. Then on the right side of the paper, reframe the thought to a neutral one. Read the reframed thoughts out loud. The positive shift is eye-opening.

Example:

<u>Negative thought</u>   <u>Reframed thought</u>

"I hate my job, I have toxic coworkers"   *"This is my job right now to support my family"*

Mindfulness enables reframing by interrupting negative automatic thoughts and allowing for more objective, conscious reflection. For example, an automatic thought, like "I'm stupid" every time you make a mistake. Making mistakes doesn't mean you are stupid, but that thought makes you feel bad. You might even believe it! Mindfulness reduces these negative thoughts. Instead of automatically thinking "I'm stupid", you can detach from the situation and adjust your perspective to "I'm glad this was a minor error and I caught it right away." No benefit comes from judging and labeling yourself.

As you reduce negative thoughts, you reduce negative emotions. Our thoughts create after-effects that can either boost us upward or push us downward if we are not mindfully aware of them.

Silence the negative self-talk

Mindfulness practice reduces negative rumination about yourself. Rumination is obsessive thinking, such as constant self-criticism. Thinking "I am not smart enough, I am not thin enough, I am not popular enough." You obsess over the negative. It's easy to fall into this mental space if you don't protect yourself through awareness.

Mindfulness halts the negative thought stream, the constant self-criticism and judgment. This positive mindset lights a path toward increasingly healthier thought patterns. The brain finds healthier circuits to follow when dealing with challenging situations. Reducing negative thought patterns unburdens the mind in a powerful way. A healthier version of you emerges.

The major impact of meta-awareness

Meta-awareness is the ability to detach from your immediate experience and be an objective observer of it. For instance, you just parked your car in the parking lot and are walking toward the store. On your way, a woman starts screaming at you because one of your tires touches the parking lot line. She is not satisfied with how you parked your car. She is hostile and aggressive, an outsized reaction given the situation. Rather than screaming back, you don't engage. You continue on your way. Think about how this shift impacts your mindset as you move on with your day. Not letting someone suck you into their toxic behavior or dysfunction; it is not your burden to carry.

Meta-awareness is when you are able to monitor and control your thoughts and emotions, as opposed to being consumed or taken over by them. You can step away from the immediate subjective experience, like that woman screaming at you for a trivial reason, to a more objective awareness. You observe her behavior and choose not to engage with it. You are less reactive and tolerate difficult situations better; it takes more to shake your composure. Meta-awareness enables the separation of emotions and thoughts from your true self; it is a superpower. The world is more clear when you exist above the chaos and the noise.

The connection between thoughts, emotions, and pain levels

Your thoughts and emotions affect how you experience pain because pain is a physical (sensory) and emotional experience. A negative emotional state increases pain, whereas a positive state lowers pain.[15]

---

[15] M. Catherine Bushnell, Marta Ceko, and Lucie A. Low, "Cognitive and Emotional Control of Pain and Its Disruption in Chronic Pain," Nature Reviews Neuroscience 14, no. 7 (July 2013): 502–11.

PAIN IS A PHYSICAL(SENSORY) AND EMOTIONAL EXPERIENCE

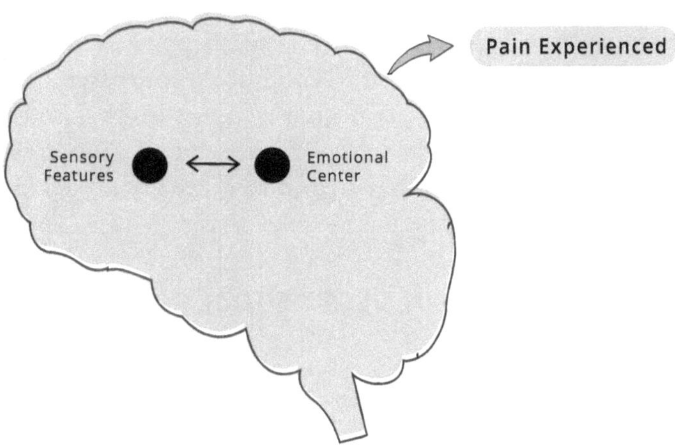

Emotions play a role in how we perceive pain because of how the brain processes it.

1. Pain is registered in the brain through multiple inputs.

2. One set of inputs reports the location and intensity of the pain.

3. Another set of inputs connects to the emotional center of the brain, called the limbic system, and reports how unpleasant the pain feels.

4. From here, circuits adjust the pain signal, either increasing or decreasing it. Positive emotions decrease the signal while negative emotions increase it. Your attention state—whether you're distracted by an activity or focused on the pain—also alters how the brain processes pain.

Negative thoughts and emotions intensify pain perception. For example, if you have a headache and you are angry about a work conflict, the pain will feel worse than if you have the same headache while you're outside, enjoying the sunshine, feeling content and free. Developing awareness of negative emotions—like sadness, frustration, anger, disappointment, or resentment—helps you cope with them in a healthy way.

With mindfulness practice, you train yourself to be aware when negative thoughts and emotions are present. Halting or reframing negative thoughts reduces the pain's intensity as you develop the ability to reduce the emotional center input. This turns down the misery input in your brain.

Neurocircuitry: Let's get nerdy

Mindfulness practice can reduce perceived pain levels by up to 30 percent. Mindfulness meditation reduces the communication between the parts of the brain responsible for relaying pain information (the thalamus) and the parts that generate self-awareness (default mode network).[16] There is awareness of the self and there is awareness of the pain, but they are not mixed into one. Because they aren't working as one, the pain level is lower.

HOW MINDFULNESS REDUCES PAIN LEVELS

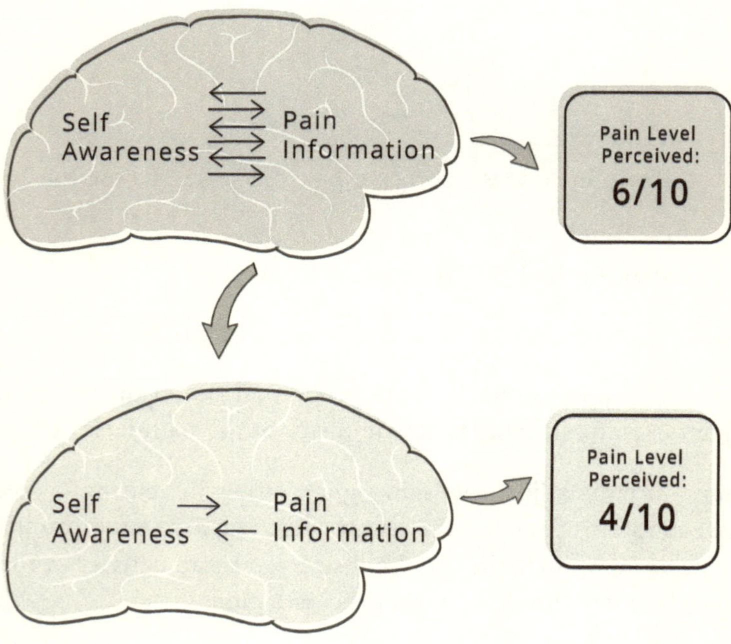

Think of this pain communication as if the self were not answering pain's phone calls, and that's a good thing! The weaker connectivity between the two areas reduces the pain you experience. Mindfulness fosters a nonreactive sense of self, which includes the experience of pain.

---

[16] Gabriel Riegner et al., "Disentangling Self from Pain: Mindfulness Meditation-induced Pain Relief is Driven by Thalamic-default Mode Network Decoupling." Pain 164, no. 2 (Feb 2023): 280-291.

──────────── **BOTTOM LINE** ────────────

Mindfulness promotes awareness of experience, without judgment, a calm observational state of being. The practice improves your ability to regulate thoughts and emotions. It fosters healthy coping through the ability to shift perspective and decrease negative thinking. With practice, it brings meta-awareness, the ability to detach from your immediate experience and be an objective observer with a controlled response. You become separate from your emotions and thoughts; your true self shines through.

CHAPTER 15

Darren's story: When stress becomes a gut punch

DARREN WAS A NICE GUY. Brown hair, lean build, good job. The ladies loved Darren. When he walked into the office, women huddled together and giggled. I witnessed it once; I have never seen such a display. Darren was oblivious with just a pinch of cluelessness.

While he was clueless about that appeal, he couldn't ignore his chronic digestive issues. Darren told me the doctor diagnosed his condition as "irritable bowel." He had seen a couple of GI doctors in the past and the work-up was negative. He had seen a functional medicine doctor who worked on nutrition and gut health, too. Yet, his digestive system was so sensitive that he could barely eat one or two meals per day. He rarely went out at night with friends because he could not tolerate eating or drinking. Everyone noticed. It was embarrassing.

We dug deeper to find the source of Darren's discomfort. Irritable bowel, yes, but what was driving it? We talked about work. He worked long hours and had a lot of responsibility, but that didn't bother him. He was capable at his work and felt good about it. In fact, he could stop working whenever he wanted; he had the financial means. So we explored life outside of work. I asked about family and relationships. He admitted he was in a relationship but was not sure it was working anymore. As we talked more about it, his stomach started hurting! As he talked more, he expanded on what a hard time he had meeting anyone. Having some mutual friends, I asked him about all the women at the office who were interested in him. And, how no fewer than three of my friends had been interested. His eyes got real big as he said "Really? I never noticed anything." Ohhh, Darren. Despite his popularity with the ladies, dating and relationships completely stressed him out.

Your GI tract has feelings, too

Since his gastrointestinal distress was so bothersome, along with irritable bowel and anxiety, I prescribed a trial of buspirone. Buspirone helps with anxiety and digestive symptoms. Darren's GI distress rating went from an eight out of ten to a four out of ten. For sensitization syndromes, such as irritable bowel, a fifty percent reduction in symptoms is a fantastic initial response. Typically, improvement in sensitization syndromes is a process that takes time, with six months being the time frame to turn down the pain level.

After weeks of contemplation, Darren moved on from his relationship. Over the next few months, his GI distress decreased. He weaned off the buspirone. Darren's mind communicated with him through his GI tract, and now, his mind was satisfied with his circumstances.

Darren continued to have multiple women asking him out at a time. He tried dating three at once, but became sick to his stomach. He listened to his body. He returned to dating one person. The last time I checked, he is eating three meals a day without a problem, so it must be going well.

The brain and gut are BFFs

Anxiety can manifest physically in the digestive tract, which includes the stomach and intestines. The digestive tract or "gut" is sensitive to your inner state and emotions. The brain and the gut have a special connection; they are BFFs.

Your brain and gut talk to each other. Do you feel butterflies in your stomach or nauseous before giving a presentation? Lose your appetite after a break-up? Darren's gut became talkative when a relationship wasn't working. These physical symptoms happen when the brain sends signals to the gut and the gut sends signals to the brain. It is a common way that our brain talks to us.

The gut is controlled by its own set of nerves called the enteric nervous system (ENS), which communicates with the brain. The brain-gut connection consists of two-way messaging between the ENS and the brain. This relationship connects the emotional and cognitive parts of the brain with gastrointestinal functions. In response to emotions or stress, the brain communicates with the intestinal tract. Having a stomachache when you are worried is an accurate message.

Cramping, diarrhea, and pain every day—such as with irritable bowel syndrome—are not accurate messages. This messaging reflects dysfunction in the brain-gut system. The dysfunction results in hypersensitivity (pain and discomfort) and changes in motility (e.g., diarrhea and constipation).

BRAIN - GUT AXIS

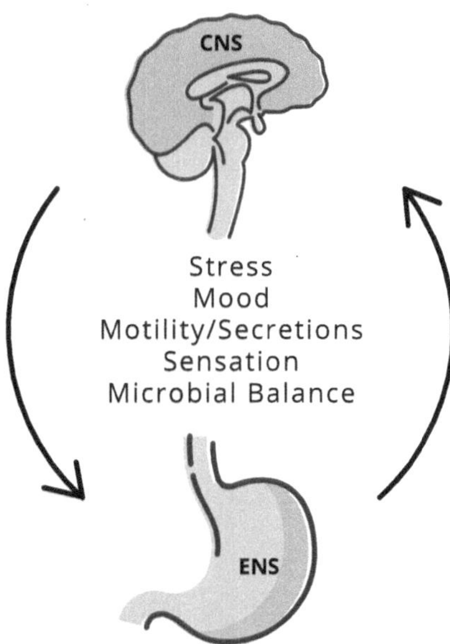

Darren's relationship stress triggered stomach troubles. His stomach and heart—emotions, to be exact—talk to each other. Sometimes, they shout.

He used awareness to understand and manage the symptoms. When eating leads to pain, he looks at his relationship. His body tells him when the relationship is not working. Darren remains off of buspirone; his symptoms improved after he resolved the emotional stress.

--- BOTTOM LINE ---

Stress likes to speak through your digestive tract. Common brain-gut symptoms are stomach pain, heartburn, and diarrhea. The brain-gut system can develop dysfunction resulting in disorders like irritable bowel syndrome or chronic stomach pain.

Your psychological state truly affects your physical state. Your body screams at you when stressed. The question is, are you going to listen? I wish I had.

CHAPTER 16

Sometimes, you need some help: Medical therapy for nerve and sensitization pain

I'VE SPENT A LOT OF time explaining sensitization. You know that it's a difficult condition to diagnose. Awareness is critical in taking positive steps. But understanding sensitization and strengthening the mind-body connection are not always enough. If the nervous system is misfiring, medical therapy to calm and reset the nerves is helpful. Medications that help sensitization pain are in the same group that helps nerve pain. Makes sense, since both pain types involve problems in the nervous system.

Three classes of medications help with relieving nerve and sensitization pain. They are called "neuropathic agents" and are classified into three categories: anticonvulsants, tricyclics, and SNRIs (serotonin and norepinephrine reuptake inhibitors). These medications were originally developed for other medical conditions, but found to reduce nerve and sensitization pain. The anticonvulsants were developed for seizures, the tricyclics for depression, and SNRIs for depression and anxiety.

Going off-label

Off-label refers to using a medication for a condition not rubber-stamped by the FDA. That doesn't mean it's unsafe or ineffective. Not every drug can get labeled for every condition, especially medications for symptom management.

For example, let's say one hundred medical conditions cause nerve pain. A new medication is developed that helps nerve pain. It's unlikely all one hundred conditions will be studied to see if the new medication helps each one. Instead, it will be labeled for a couple of the conditions and made available for off-label use.

Is this a safe practice?

Off-label use is common for sensitization syndromes, rare conditions, and medical conditions that don't generate money. If there is no money to be made, the incentive and ability to study the condition is lower. Studies are expensive and resource-intensive. Still, people with these conditions need help and symptom relief. Off-label use allows providers to prescribe a medication for a medical condition for which there would otherwise be no treatment option. Also, the medications selected as off-label either have studies supporting their use or target the same dysfunction the medication was designed for. I say this to clarify that off-label use is not as scandalous as it sounds.

Anticonvulsants– gabapentin, pregabalin, lamotrigine, oxcarbazepine

The first class of medications is the anticonvulsant class. These medications are FDA-approved to treat seizures, but have also been shown to work for treating nerve pain. These meds lower nerve excitability, which reduces seizures and also reduces pain signals, so you feel less pain. Anticonvulsants turn down the volume of the pain. For example, if your sensitization pain is rated as eight out of ten, a neuropathic agent may lower it to four.

Although FDA-approved for seizures, gabapentin and pregabalin are better suited for treating nerve pain. This class is generally the first-line medical therapy for acute nerve pain, like sciatica or pinched nerves. Anticonvulsants are also effective for treating chronic nerve pain. For harder to treat cases or if another medication is needed, oxcarbazepine and lamotrigine have research that supports their effectiveness, too.

Tricyclics– amitriptyline, nortriptyline

The second class of neuropathic medications is the tricyclics, which include amitriptyline and nortriptyline. They have been around for sixty years. They are inexpensive and effective at low doses. Although FDA-labeled to treat depression, tricyclics are now used more often to treat a variety of pain conditions.

Ample evidence supports the use of amitriptyline for multiple sensitization syndromes and nerve pain.[17] They include fibromyalgia, headaches, irritable

---

[17] Accessed on May 4, 2023. https://www.micromedexsolutions.com/home/dispatch

bowel syndrome, and neuropathy. Tricyclics are also helpful for sleep, a useful benefit because nerve pain feels worse at night, interfering with sleep.

Tricyclics do have side effects that limit their use. In particular, tricyclics are not a good choice for people who have heart disease, multiple medical issues, decreased memory, or for older adults.

SNRIs (serotonin and norepinephrine reuptake inhibitors)– duloxetine, venlafaxine

The third class of neuropathic agents is the SNRIs. They increase the amount of serotonin and norepinephrine in the brain—messengers that help with mood and pain. A common example is duloxetine. It is FDA-approved for the treatment of multiple types of chronic pain, depression, and anxiety. An SNRI is a good choice for someone who needs treatment for depression, anxiety, sensitization, or nerve pain. Venlafaxine is also in this class and should theoretically help with pain. In my clinical experience, I didn't see venlafaxine as an effective treatment for nerve pain.

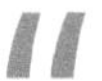

> MEDICAL THERAPY FOR SENSITIZATION-
> RELATED PAIN IS NOT STRAIGHTFORWARD.
> ONE SIZE FITS NO ONE.

Sensitization—Nerve pain management 101

Each person has their own effective medication and their own effective dose. Some need low doses for relief, while others need higher doses. Because of this variability, adequate titration is key to finding relief. Medication titration is the process of adjusting the dose upward until you find the maximum benefit or until side effects limit its use.

A common reason patients came to see me was because of ineffective pain control. Typically, the problem was either the wrong medication for the pain type (using anti-inflammatory medications for nerve pain) or the medication dose was not titrated properly. For example, Linda suffered from sciatic nerve pain in her back and leg. She had seen a provider for the pain and they prescribed gabapentin. She told me gabapentin didn't work. I asked her what the dose was. She said one hundred milligrams. I increased Linda's dose to three hundred milligrams and her pain level improved substantially. It wasn't that the medication did not work for her; the issue was inadequate titration. Your body chemistry is unique, so work with your provider to find the right medication at the right dosage.

Which works best for me?

Each medication class lowers pain through a different way. The class that works best for you depends on your body chemistry and your combination of symptoms. Using one medication to treat multiple symptoms is ideal because it reduces the number of medications and reduces side effects. For example, if you have nerve pain AND you can't sleep at night, a medication that calms nerve signals and aids sleep is a good fit. The anticonvulsant and tricyclic classes both help with nerve pain and sleep. Alternatively, if you're suffering from nerve pain and depression, the SNRI class may be best. The least amount of medical therapy to alleviate suffering is the goal.

More relief options

Acupuncture is a non-medication option for nerve and sensitization pain. It is an Eastern medical therapy that inserts tiny needles in specific points in the body to bring balance to the nervous system. Acupuncture may be used alone or in combination with medical therapy for a variety of sensitization syndromes such as migraines, back pain, irritable bowel, and fibromyalgia.

Nerve stimulators come in a variety of different types and may blunt nerve and sensitization pain. They range from the TENS unit (transcutaneous electrical nerve stimulation) that you place on the outside of your body to spinal cord stimulators that are surgically placed inside your body. The research and feedback I have received regarding how well these devices work varies from not helping at all to moderate help. Talk with your provider or physical therapist about whether a trial of nerve stimulation is an option to consider.

Cannabinoids are a group of substances found in the cannabis plant. Two well-known cannabinoids are THC and cannabidiol (CBD). Cannabidiol is another option for treating sensitization pain. When I worked in the multiple sclerosis clinic, many patients found CBD helpful for nerve pain, especially when it flared at night. It also reduced muscle spasms and promoted sleep. Using CBD drops before bed is a common regimen. And unlike THC, CBD promotes brain health rather than hurts it.[18]

---

[18] Albert Batalla et al., "The Impact of Cannabidiol on Human Brain Function: A Systematic Review," *Frontiers in Pharmacology* 11 (January 2021). https://doi.org/10.3389/fphar.2020.618184.

Low-dose naltrexone (LDN) has shown promise for reducing chronic pain in sensitization syndromes. LDN may help by decreasing inflammation in the nervous system.

Alpha-lipoic acid[19] and **Acetyl-L-carnitine**[20] are over-the-counter supplements that potentially deliver benefits for nerve pain.

Topical options for nerve pain relief include lidocaine patches and capsaicin patches. Some multiple sclerosis patients found lidocaine patches helpful for severe nerve pain in their legs and feet.

Low-dose ketamine, an anesthetic agent, is an emerging treatment for nerve and sensitization pain. Ketamine is a consideration when first, second, and third line medications have failed. Recent studies show promise of low-dose ketamine for the treatment of nerve-like pain and severe depression. Scientists are currently evaluating low-dose ketamine for sensitization syndromes, such as headaches, fibromyalgia, and low back pain.[21] To learn if ketamine is a viable option for you, consult a pain specialist. At high doses, ketamine works as an anesthetic agent, so you want a doctor specialized and knowledgeable in its use.

Psychedelics are gaining interest for their potential use for the treatment of chronic pain with the theory they may be able to reset the misfiring neural pathways.[22] Psychedelics, such as psilocybin, are also being studied with new dosing regimens for difficult to treat depression or treatment resistant depression.[23]

---

[19] Dan Ziegler et al., "Efficacy and Safety of Antioxidant Treatment with Alpha-lipoic Acid Over 4 Years in Diabetic Polyneuropathy: the NATHAN 1 Trial," Diabetes Care 34, no. 9 (September 2011): 2054-60.

[20] Anders AF Sima et al., "Acetyl-L-carnitine Improves Pain, Nerve Regeneration, and Vibratory Perception in Patients with Chronic Diabetic Neuropathy: An Analysis of Two Randomized Placebo-controlled Trials," Diabetes Care, 28, no. 1 (January 2005): 89-94.

[21] Steven P. Cohen et al., "Consensus Guidelines on the Use of Intravenous Ketamine Infusions for Chronic Pain From the American Society of Regional Anesthesia and Pain Medicine, the American Academy of Pain Medicine, and the American Society of Anesthesiologists," Regional Anesthesia and Pain Medicine 43, no. 5 (July 2018): 521-546. https://doi.org/10.1097/aap.0000000000000808.

[22] Joel P. Castellanos et al., "Chronic Pain and Psychedelics: A Review and Proposed Mechanism of Action," Regional Anesthesia and Pain Medicine 45, no. 7 (May 2020): 486–494. https://doi.org/10.1136/rapm-2020-101273.

[23] Guy M. Goodwin et al., "Single-Dose Psilocybin for a Treatment-Resistant Episode of Major Depression," New England Journal of Medicine 387 (November 2022): 1637–1648. https://doi.org/10.1056/nejmoa2206443.

Depression can creep in and change the mindset. Depression makes the world appear in shades of gray, as happiness and color are lost. Thinking becomes negative and rigid. Purpose is lost. Psilocybin helps people break out of this mindset.[24]

BOTTOM LINE

Medical therapy is useful to calm over-reactive nerves and reduce pain levels from nerve sensitization. There are three main categories of medications that lower nerve pain: anticonvulsants, tricyclics, and SNRIs. Other options include acupuncture and cannabidiol, which help with nerve pain, muscle spasm, and sleep. Emerging treatments include low dose ketamine and new dosing regimens of psychedelics, such as psilocybin.

Medical therapy plays an important role in chronic pain. When your pain is better managed, you can concentrate on the other aspects of healing, including building awareness, practicing mindfulness, and strengthening the mind-body connection. You can't take the steps towards healing if you are consumed by pain! You are just trying to survive in that state. Just remember that the actual medication and dosage needs to be tailored to you. Although there can be a frustrating trial-and-error period when seeking the right fit, when you find it, it is a life-changer. You get your life back.

---

[24] Richard E. Daws et al., "Increased Global Integration in the Brain after Psilocybin Therapy for Depression," Nature Medicine 28 (April 2022): 844–51. https://doi.org/10.1038/s41591-022-01744-z.

CHAPTER 17

Stress Rx on the treatment note

THE NEGATIVE IMPACT OF STRESS on our health is not a new concept. Yet, in my experience, few people or providers understand or address the role that stress plays in medical conditions. We know how lifting or repetitive motion can cause injuries. We understand that air and water quality can affect our health. But when it comes to stress or trauma as a cause for poor health, we don't seem to have space on our treatment note for it. At best, it is unacknowledged. At worst, there is no awareness of its relationship to treatment.

After my time working in the clinic, I transitioned to working with the Medicaid program. I was going to help fix the healthcare system. My naïveté was almost as overblown as my past denial. Turns out there are a lot of politics involved in how the healthcare system operates! The political opposition to change made the process feel like walking through mud. Thick, boot-sucking mud with your feet stuck two feet deep. I saw first-hand the issues with special interest groups. The people getting rich off the current system don't want the system to change. And they are the ones with money and influence to prevent it.

Good studies, bad studies

My main role with the Medicaid program was to develop medical policy. I reviewed science papers about emerging medical treatments to determine if the studies supported that the therapies were effective. If the studies supported effectiveness, I would draft a medical policy and include it in the Medicaid program. If the studies did not support it, the therapy would not be covered by the program.

During this time, my supervising physician was Oxford-trained in evidence-based medicine—possessing the skill of being able to analyze and understand which research studies can be believed (yes, not every positive study means the treatment works). Poorly designed studies can use smoke and mirrors to create an illusion of benefit. And the company can make a lot of money during the five- to ten-year period it takes for the smoke to clear and people to notice it doesn't work.

Skills in evidence-based medicine allow you to see the studies with real results, versus the ones that have been designed for a positive result to sell a therapy. Spoiler alert, a lot of pain cures and arthritis treatments are just that. The company advertises miraculous results; yet, when you try that medication, it doesn't do much. The positive results of the studies were not real; they were illusions.

Let me stand on my soap box a bit longer. Studies can be designed to show benefits by using poor quality methods that leverage human psychology. The placebo effect is an example, if you give someone a treatment they hope will work, use a subjective outcome measure such as asking them if it works, they will report a benefit, even if it was water.

Providers have the same issue. If they know someone in a study is getting the actual treatment, they are likely to say it helped, as opposed to not knowing who in the study got the treatment and thus having no bias. That is why objective measures not based on subjective experience are important. Hope is powerful but it shouldn't be used to get people to pay for treatments that don't help. There is plenty of free snake oil for that.

Over the years I spent with the Medicaid program, I found most of the published studies that I reviewed were low quality and the results could not be believed! That is why the quality of the study is critically important when reviewing the results. It is easy to be fooled.

This kind of discrepancy in study quality is why we see promising therapies with initial positive results later turn out to be ineffective. Early studies are small with poor quality but promising, a sign to study in greater detail and not end it there. Later, when higher quality studies are done—eliminating bias— the benefit may disappear or it can be verified. We saw this with hydroxychloroquine during the covid pandemic. Early studies showed promise. With further higher quality studies, the benefit faded away. I spent a lot of time discussing this nuance with doctors who felt any positive study meant a treatment is effective. Not true at all. Do a study poorly enough and you can show a treatment effect. Just not an accurate one.

From proof to policy

Anyway, if the treatment met the efficacy and safety standards of Washington state, then it was my job to draft a medical policy. The medical policy described under what criteria the treatment would be covered as part of the Medicaid benefit. For example, back surgery has a medical policy. Studies support when back surgeries tend to help, when they don't, and when they cause harm. Back surgery has a unique safety concern because a significant percentage of people have more pain and disability after the back surgery. I am familiar with this group because these surgical patients ended up in my clinic for chronic pain management following unsuccessful surgeries. There is even a billing code for it, "failed back surgery syndrome". The medical policy details the screens that determine who may benefit and who may worsen. Well, that was the idea. I obtained feedback on the policy draft from top specialists in an area as part of the process. It was a positive, collaborative effort ninety percent of the time.

Over the years, I observed when a surgery or procedure pays a large sum of money, it tended to be overused. By overused, I mean offered to people who don't need it or are not good candidates for the procedure. This issue was rampant for spinal injections and back surgery during this time period.

To minimize the excessive use of certain treatments, another part of my job was to review procedure requests for specific patients to see if the person planned for the procedure met the criteria for whom the procedure was helpful or check for a justifiable exception. Clinical medicine is shades of gray—not black and white—especially with pain syndromes. Ninety percent of medical practices do the right thing, the process I'm describing is for the ten percent that don't.

In fairness, I also saw the insurance companies abuse this process, denying procedures that fell into the gray area to save money or because the staff hired to review the procedure requests didn't have the training or expertise to review the request accurately. This process tortured the surgeons as they had to take time and explain to a non-physician why a complicated patient needed a procedure. It was a mess.

Stress and trauma didn't qualify for the clinic note

I spent a considerable amount of time reviewing medical records and treatment plans for various medical conditions, including chronic back pain, chronic headaches, chronic digestive issues, and chronic bladder pain.

" UNDERSTANDING THE ROLE OF STRESS, TRAUMA, AND SENSITIZATION IS CRITICAL TO SUCCESSFUL TREATMENT. "

Conditions where understanding the role of stress, trauma, and sensitization is critical to successful treatment. Yet, the role of these contributing factors was rarely mentioned or addressed in the documentation I received. The contribution of sensitization to the symptoms was rarely noted.

I recall reviewing charts of women with chronic bladder pain, interstitial cystitis—a diagnosis that frequently carries a pertinent history of severe childhood trauma, particularly sexual abuse. However, the medical record documentation I reviewed infrequently included information about past trauma. Come to think of it, I don't recall one that did. Instead, I saw notes about procedure after procedure being performed with minimal benefit. I had to review the chart because the provider had requested yet another procedure after a slew of those that delivered no effect. Meanwhile, the catalyst of the condition was not mentioned in the treatment plan. The patient wasn't even asked about factors like childhood trauma. Yes, the subject is a big issue to address in a ten-minute clinic visit, but ignoring the issue misses a critical piece relevant to treatment.

I sent Bryan to a neurologist for a second opinion on his stress-induced migraines. After doing so, he reported there was not one question or discussion about the role stress played in his headaches starting or continuing. They confirmed the diagnosis and recommended he increase the medication dose. Stress was the root cause of his headaches and the trigger for headache flares and it was not even mentioned.

In my experience, the traditional medical model does not address the role of stress or trauma in triggering and worsening medical disorders (beyond a psychological referral that is disconnected from the medical treatment). In medical training and my personal experience, evaluating a patient's symptoms prioritized looking for a tumor, infection, or circulation problem. If those were not found, the person was ok. But, the source of disabling physical symptoms is ordinarily not a tumor or infection. The issue is something we cannot see or measure.

Stress-related disorders, like headaches, digestive issues, and pain interfere with people's ability to work, support themselves, and care for their family. These effects turn into feelings of shame, loss of purpose, and social isolation. A negative spiral of greater and greater loss ensues. In my experience, medications or procedures were offered but the underlying cause was rarely pursued or addressed. The most effective treatments were seldom discussed.

When you don't connect how stress or past trauma is making you sick or contributing to your symptoms, how can you take action to heal? If I hadn't figured out that my stomach pain was related to stress, I would not have known to make the needed changes to regain my health. Awareness of the cause is the stimulus for the actions needed to heal. As providers, we should help people make that connection.

There is ample scientific evidence supporting the medical basis for these disorders and their holistic treatment approach. Complicating matters is the fact that the current healthcare payer system makes it difficult for providers to apply. Almost impossible. Find the lesion, do a procedure, next patient. That is the clinic model that is financially sustainable, but it is not the correct treatment for these disorders. Fixing this medical payer model has proven insurmountable to date. The groups getting rich off the current system don't want the system to change. Special interests...don't get me started.

I didn't make much progress rehabilitating the medical system during my time with the Medicaid program. Even the legislators I met with seemed deflated, drained, and defeated by the topic.

BOTTOM LINE

Stress-related disorders—like headaches, digestive issues, and pain—rob people of their lives; constant suffering takes its toll. Despite the role that stress plays in these disorders, in my experience, it is rarely considered in their treatment. Since understanding the role of stress and trauma is critical for healing, I hope having the conversation here will help you. Awareness is the catalyst for effective action and healing.

CHAPTER 18

Kristina's story: The slow creep of clinical depression

KRISTINA WAS THIRTY-TWO YEARS OLD, tall, thin, and Ivy League-educated. She showed exceptional talent in everything she did. Not only a capable administrator, but also an accomplished writer and musician—and she was nice, too. Kristina's perceivable flaw was her addiction to pleasing the people around her.

She worked on public health projects, managing teams of people and moving progress along, like new medical benefits and care programs. With the completion of each project, Kristina would scan the room for approving eyes. Then, she'd listen attentively for people's positive feedback about what a stellar job she did. Generally, she received the positive reaction she craved.

But all was not well with Kristina. On the outside, she presented with a big smile. If you looked closely, you could see sadness in her eyes. As Kristina started on the next work project, unusual thoughts crept into her head. At first, a few times a week, she would introspectively question herself and her work.

"What's the point?"

"Does this matter?"

As the weeks wore on, she became increasingly indifferent towards work. At times, Kristina didn't even look for colleague's approval.

The thoughts started popping into her head more. Daily, she wondered,

"Why am I doing this?"

Kristina continued to report to work and appear engaged, but she wasn't. She politely accepted requests with a smile. Then, she looked away as her smile languished.

On her calendar, she noted a cooking class. Kristina had been waiting for months to try it. Now, she didn't care. She headed home to rest. Her stomach ached.

Later that week, Kristina's friends invited her out for drinks. She passed. She wanted to go home and rest. Besides, her stomach hurt.

Over a matter of months, Kristina lost interest in her job, lost interest in her hobbies, and lost interest in spending time with friends. She felt utterly indifferent to the world around her. There did not seem to be a point to anything. Her mindset had changed.

Kristina didn't feel like herself and had a nagging stomachache. She made an appointment to check in with her doctor.

Her doctor asked, "Have you lost interest in things that you used to do for fun?"

Kristina replied, "Well, I have lost interest in my work, but maybe I need a new job. I guess I also stopped doing some other things too, like my cooking class."

"Are you feeling down or sad?"

She replied, "I just don't see the point of things. I am not crying or anything."

"Any trouble with sleep?"

She replied, "I sleep a lot, but then I still feel tired."

Her doctor paused. Kristina looked ok. She was high functioning with good work performance. She had friends. From the outside, Kristina looked ok. From the inside, it's a different view. The widespread disinterest, fatigue, excessive sleeping, and stomach pain are suggestive of clinical depression. A depression Kristina was unaware of. Sure, she lost interest in work and cooking but she wasn't lying in bed all day or crying frequently. Her depression didn't present like that.

A prominent feature of Kristina's depression is a symptom known as "anhedonia". Anhedonia is a lack of interest or indifference to activities once enjoyed. It can progress to not seeing the point in anything, to not seeing the point in living. And, tragically, to feeling that your loved ones are better off without you.

The depression mindset slowly overtook Kristina's thought patterns. The depressed thoughts felt rational, logical. They were a subtle, invisible creep.

Sometimes, even those suffering from anhedonia aren't aware of the situation. Those around them see a person who appears to be functioning well. These are the people who look fine on the outside and then you hear they died by suicide. Severe depression is easily missed in cases like Kristina's.

CHAPTER 19

Depression doesn't look depressed

DEPRESSION PRESENTS IN MANY DIFFERENT and unexpected ways. The condition is categorized as a psychological disorder; however, it presents with both psychological and physical symptoms. Commonly reported psychological symptoms include low mood and loss of interest. Sometimes, the physical symptoms are the main indicators. In the **DEPRESS II** study,[25] two of the three most common symptoms reported during a depressive episode were physical. They included having no energy/feeling tired (73 percent) and broken/decreased sleep (63 percent). It is not just the mind that is depressed, but the whole body that slows down.

Depression doesn't look like you might expect. You might imagine someone with clinical depression acts somber. Someone walking around with their head down and a tear in their eye. Or someone who can't get out of bed in the morning. Sometimes, that is the case.

Oftentimes, a depressed person looks like Kristina. They appear fine on the outside, while a cloud of despair looms on the inside. Kristina experienced complete indifference (anhedonia), fatigue, and sleep changes. She appeared fine to her coworkers and friends, despite worsening depression.

Depression sneaks up on people and distorts their mindset, slowly changing what matters to them. Slowly taking away all that matters. As we saw with

---

[25] André Tylee and Paul Gandhi, "The Importance of Somatic Symptoms in Depression in Primary Care," The Primary Care Companion J Clin Psychiatry 7, no. 4 (2005): 167-176.

Kristina, she went from being motivated and engaged in her work to seeing no purpose in it. Her passion for cooking evaporated. Valuing time with her friends slipped away as she preferred hanging out alone. Nothing about work or life had changed. Kristina's mindset had changed.

Kristina's story of depression demonstrates how severe depression goes unnoticed. Despite how much she struggled on the inside, Kristina performed well at work and appeared normal. Like many medical issues with the brain, the struggle is invisible from the outside. The internal suffering can't be seen. When someone has a stroke and can't walk, the physical signs are obvious. Unfortunately, with brain disorders, like depression, the signs cannot be seen. We can't understand or assess their experience by what we see on the outside. The changes to how their brain works are not apparent. We can learn about the view from the inside. With this work, we can reduce how often we hear after a death from depression or suicide, "there were no signs of a problem."

Depression and anxiety make everything more miserable

Sensitization may bring about depression and anxiety. Conversely, depression and anxiety increase the suffering from sensitization syndromes. It's a negative feedback loop that spirals, worsening both disorders.[26]

People struggling with depression or anxiety may not be aware of it, especially if the symptoms are mostly physical. For instance, I had a patient cry throughout a clinic visit, reporting she could not get out of bed each day and would cry multiple times per week, but still denied being sad or upset. I have had people trembling from anxiety or having a panic attack in front of me who tell me they are not anxious. The diagnosis is not as obvious as you might think. And, it can be difficult to see in yourself.

Since depression presents with diverse combinations of psychological and physical symptoms, providers use clinical measures or tools to increase awareness of it. You can use these tools too. With improved awareness, you can better advocate for yourself when you talk with your provider.

The patient health questionnaire 9 (**PHQ**-9) is useful for checking depression symptoms and is used by primary care providers. The tool provides a detached view of how you are feeling. The **PHQ**-9 poses questions about common signs of depression, such as feeling down and loss of interest in doing things. It also covers the common physical symptoms of depression, like low energy and disrupted sleep.

---

[26] Leah M. Adams and Dennis C. Turk, "Psychosocial Factors and Central Sensitivity Syndromes," Current Rheumatology Reviews 11, no. 2 (2015): 96–108. https://doi.org/1 0.2174/1573397111666150619095330.

PATIENT HEALTH QUESTIONNAIRE-9
(PHQ-9)

Over the <u>last 2 weeks</u>, how often have you been bothered by any of the following problems? *(Use "✔" to indicate your answer)*	Not at all	Several days	More than half the days	Nearly every day
1. Little interest or pleasure in doing things	0	1	2	3
2. Feeling down, depressed, or hopeless	0	1	2	3
3. Trouble falling or staying asleep, or sleeping too much	0	1	2	3
4. Feeling tired or having little energy	0	1	2	3
5. Poor appetite or overeating	0	1	2	3
6. Feeling bad about yourself — or that you are a failure or have let yourself or your family down	0	1	2	3
7. Trouble concentrating on things, such as reading the newspaper or watching television	0	1	2	3
8. Moving or speaking so slowly that other people could have noticed? Or the opposite — being so fidgety or restless that you have been moving around a lot more than usual	0	1	2	3
9. Thoughts that you would be better off dead or of hurting yourself in some way	0	1	2	3

FOR OFFICE CODING ___0___ + _______ + _______ + _______

=Total Score: _______

If you checked off <u>any</u> problems, how <u>difficult</u> have these problems made it for you to do your work, take care of things at home, or get along with other people?

Not difficult at all	Somewhat difficult	Very difficult	Extremely difficult
☐	☐	☐	☐

Developed by Drs. Robert L. Spitzer, Janet B.W. Williams, Kurt Kroenke and colleagues, with an educational grant from Pfizer Inc. No permission required to reproduce, translate, display or distribute.

The PHQ-9 score is calculated by assigning scores of zero, one, two, or three to the responses ranging from "not at all" to "nearly every day." After answering the questions, your total score is calculated within a range from zero to twenty-seven. A score of ten or more suggests moderate depression symptoms, while a score of twenty or more suggests severe symptoms. This rating scale can also be used periodically to follow the severity of symptoms over time.

The PHQ-9 is a tool for improving awareness of depression symptoms. By itself, the questionnaire should not be used for diagnosis. A complete clinical picture is required for an accurate diagnosis and the PHQ-9 does not provide that. For example, the PHQ-9 does not check for other medical conditions that can cause symptoms similar to depression, such as low thyroid. Nor does it check for other mental health conditions, such as bipolar disorder, which can present similar to depression but requires different treatment.

Warning signs: Your body is sending an alert

We discussed earlier how depression presents with both psychological and physical symptoms. Psychological symptoms include low mood, loss of interest, and feeling badly about yourself. For some, physical symptoms—like fatigue and sleep changes—are more evident. There can be other physical symptoms too, such as headaches, stomach pain, and back pain, so we use another tool to help with the assessment of physical symptoms from mental health conditions.

The PHQ-15 is used to evaluate physical symptoms that may be related to a mental health condition, known clinically as "somatization". The scale helps assess the severity of the physical symptoms. As part of this process, the provider considers whether there's a separate medical issue before concluding that symptoms are solely from depression or anxiety. Frequently, there is a mix of both, with one worsening the other. For example, someone has mild back arthritis but, when experiencing depression, the pain feels worse.

Suspicion for somatization arises when there is no other biologic explanation for the physical symptoms. This situation is common, yet rarely discussed. People go down a long diagnostic journey of tests looking for a source. They're told the results came back negative and everything looks ok, so they are dismissed. The explanation that the source of the symptoms is an expression of depression or anxiety or stress is not common based on my experience. Providers have a hard time explaining somatization since the concept of how it happens in the body is poorly understood. The mind-body connection is well-documented but not well-understood. Providers fear the patient will misunderstand what they are saying and get angry. And, sometimes, the provider doesn't make the connection themselves.

PHYSICAL SYMPTOMS
(PHQ-15)

During the <u>past 4 weeks</u>, how much have you been bothered by any of the following problems?

	Not bothered at all (0)	Bothered a little (1)	Bothered a lot (2)
a. Stomach pain	☐	☐	☐
b. Back pain	☐	☐	☐
c. Pain in your arms, legs, or joints (knees, hips, etc.)	☐	☐	☐
d. Menstrual cramps or other problems with your periods **WOMEN ONLY**	☐	☐	☐
e. Headaches	☐	☐	☐
f. Chest pain	☐	☐	☐
g. Dizziness	☐	☐	☐
h. Fainting spells	☐	☐	☐
i. Feeling your heart pound or race	☐	☐	☐
j. Shortness of breath	☐	☐	☐
k. Pain or problems during sexual intercourse	☐	☐	☐
l. Constipation, loose bowels, or diarrhea	☐	☐	☐
m. Nausea, gas, or indigestion	☐	☐	☐
n. Feeling tired or having low energy	☐	☐	☐
o. Trouble sleeping	☐	☐	☐

(For office coding: Total Score T_____ = _____ + _____)

The **PHQ**-15 lists physical symptoms reported along with depression and anxiety. Various types of pain are common, including headaches, back pain, and stomach pain. The **PHQ**-15 score is calculated by assigning scores of zero, one, or two, to each of the responses, ranging from "not bothered at all" to "bothered a lot". After answering the questions, your total score is calculated. A total score of ten or more suggests medium physical symptom severity; a score of fifteen or more suggests high symptom severity.

Kristina's stomach pain is an example of somatization. She had clinical symptoms of disinterest, fatigue, and excessive sleeping. These symptoms were suggestive of major depression. She also had stomach pain. There was no other medical explanation for her stomach pain. No stomach ulcers. No gallbladder issues. Having ruled out the other medical causes for stomach pain, depression was determined to be the source. Kristina's depression improved with treatment, so did her stomach pain.

Her treatment consisted of cognitive behavioral therapy, to identify and reduce unhealthy thought patterns. For example, catching automatic negative thoughts and replacing them with more objective, positive ones. Not allowing thoughts like "I am dumb," instead replacing it with an accurate thought like "I made a minor mistake. I am learning a new skill and making mistakes is part of the learning process."

She also started medication therapy with venlafaxine, which increases the level of mood-enhancing neurotransmitters in the brain, like serotonin. Kristina's body created a physical signal to tell her she needed help. The mind-body connection at work.

BOTTOM LINE

Depression presents in various ways and creeps up slowly, invisible to the outside world. The symptoms of depression include both physical and psychological signs. The physical symptoms, like fatigue and poor sleep, may be the most apparent. Given depression's unique presentation in each individual, clinical tools are useful to check for it. The **PHQ**-9 checks for depression symptoms and the **PHQ**-15 evaluates for physical signs. Depression co-occurs with sensitization syndromes, making its identification and treatment part of treating stress-related disorders.

CHAPTER 20

Voula's story: The grown-up pain of childhood trauma

TO THIS POINT, I'VE SHARED real-life stories about people who developed painful conditions as a result of extreme stress. Stress and its impact show up in many forms. In addition to pain and digestive problems, stress can lead to mental health conditions, like anxiety and depression. And even experiences that seem buried in your past can return and wreak havoc.

One death, a lifetime of panic

Voula was 10 years old in July of 1984, hanging out with her family on the beach in Kalamata, Greece. One event was about to change her life and love for the bright blue waters forever. She loved swimming in the deep waters. Her mother often screamed, "Come closer in! Not so far!" After what happened that day, her mother's warning would never be needed. This sunny day by the beach would bring darkness to her life for years to come.

Sunning under the bright, blue sky, Voula noticed people gathering around a man near the edge of the water. They struggled to pull him to shore. He had blue swim trunks and gray hair. His body was limp. His face, pale. As they lifted him onto the beach, one of the helpers turned around and screamed, "He is not breathing! We need help." A nearby woman raced over and began chest compressions. Voula stood by helplessly, wishing she could assist.

As she watched the chest compressions, water started bubbling out of the man's mouth. His skin and body took on a blue hue. Voula's mother tried to pull her away but she couldn't move. She desperately needed to be sure the man was ok.

After what felt like an hour, but was really ten minutes, the ambulance arrived and transported him to the hospital.

Later that night, Voula and her family watched the news. They saw a report of an adult male who had drowned on the east side of Kalamata beach. She knew that it was the man she had seen earlier in the day. Voula began gasping for air, feeling lightheaded and out of breath. The young girl thought she was dying. Voula's mother splashed water on her face and laid her in bed. She gently guided her to breathe slowly and calm down.

This was Voula's first panic attack. At any age, it's scary, but when you're only ten years old, unaccustomed to life's tragedies, a panic attack can be life-changing. After that day, Voula could not go in the water past where her toes touched. If she couldn't feel the sand beneath her feet, her heart started racing and she struggled to breathe.

Voula's mother took her to a pediatrician for help with overcoming anxiety. The doctor said, "Oh, it's nothing. I can prescribe some antidepressants and she will be fine."

Her mother didn't think that she needed medication. Instead, she took Voula to their local church for a blessing from the priest.

There's no vacation from panic attacks

Voula's panic attacks continued to intensify over the next year. She tried to go to summer camp. As she sat in a circle around the campfire with the other campers, out of nowhere, she started gasping for air. She awoke in the middle of the night crying from night terrors. The camp staff, at a loss of how to help this girl, called her mother to pick her up.

After a year of unpredictable panic attacks, the episodes finally started to abate. Voula recalls a day in the park when she felt a calm come over her. The panic waned. She was herself again.

Earth-shattering experiences

Her calm was short-lived. On September 13th, 1986, Voula's mother insisted the family go to church. It was the night before the celebration of Voula's name day, a tradition in Greek culture where the origin of a person's name is celebrated. Voula's was the day of the cross. As the family entered the church, lighted charcoal and scented candles surrounded them. A smoky, incense filled the air. Voula found it hard to breathe.

The walls started closing in around her, her anxiety level began to rise. She asked her mother if she could go to the bathroom. After she approved, Voula sneaked outside for fresh air. She took a deep breath and looked at the nearby monastery cells.

As Voula inhaled the fresh air, she heard what sounded like an airplane coming in for a landing above her; a deafening rumble. She lost her footing as the ground started to shake beneath her feet. Was this the apocalypse? Had lying about using the bathroom to get out of church started it?

Just then, people started exiting the church. As they walked, they chanted "Jesus, save your people!" They continued the church service outdoors, hoping to be saved, as the earthquake broke the buildings around them into pieces. Thirty percent of the homes in the town were lost that day.

Voula's family hiked from the church through the rubble to see if their house was still standing. Although damaged, it withstood and was safe to live in. Other than the loss of electricity, they still had a home, unlike many families nearby.

Two days later, Voula was sitting outside her home, under the balcony in a wicker chair when she heard a familiar sound. The rumbling returned. She jumped out of her chair and sprinted toward St. George church. Halfway there, she realized her mother, sister and brother were still inside their house. Voula turned around and started running back toward the house when she was hit in the shoulder by a flying brick. The brick knocked her to the ground. As she raised her head to get up, Voula saw the surrounding homes bending and closing in and out. Another earthquake.

In an instant, she couldn't breathe. She gasped for air. Voula felt like she was drowning, her face and mouth smothered by dust. When the ground stopped shaking, she crawled up and headed back home. As she neared the house, she spotted the legs of the wicker chair poking out from under debris. The chair had been crushed by the balcony, which had collapsed. Their home didn't survive this earthquake. Luckily, her family did.

A life on the move

Homeless, Voula's family initially stayed with an uncle. After a few months, a local philanthropist sent a cruise ship to house the homeless. They were provided a single cabin for the family.

Voula's panic attacks returned with the earthquakes. The anxiety, fear of dying, and nightmares played in her head. She fell inside herself. Quiet, reclusive, and in shock, she spent her time praying, playing sports, and studying. She journaled every day, starting with "God, give me strength."

After living on the ship, the family transitioned to a mobile home. Voula switched schools four times that year. When they found their final spot, they began building a new home. After school, Voula helped, painting and carrying bricks to the stone masons.

She survived. Prayer, journaling, gratitude, and living in the now got her through this traumatic time. Voula journaled about building their new house. She wrote about school exams she was nervous to take. Her sister earned a few pages, on the days she bullied Voula. She wrote of her successes, like winning basketball games. She read Socrates and studied his teachings about self-knowledge.

22 years later, the panic attacks return

Fast forward 22 years later, to when Voula lived in Chicago, working through her doctoral dissertation on adult education. She hadn't been able to visit her family in Greece for three years. Recently, her mother's health had begun to fail. She had Alzheimer's and lost more of herself each day. Voula felt trapped and torn between her studies and her family.

Driving in rush hour traffic one day, she found herself gasping for air. The drowning sensation rushed over her, this time in a sea of cars. She gripped the steering wheel, her hands sweating, her heart racing. Voula managed to call a friend, who shouted, "Don't call me! Call 911! You're having a heart attack!"

The paramedics arrived to transport Voula to the hospital. As they lifted her into the ambulance, she squeaked out, "Will I be able to finish my dissertation?"

At the hospital, Voula underwent a heart work-up. As she waited for the results, an episode of "Frasier" played on the television. Coincidentally, on the show, the anxious character Niles was having trouble breathing, and Voula instantly recognized the panic attack signs in him. When the doctor came in with her test results, she learned everything was normal. The doctor said everything looked ok, it was just stress, and she could go home.

The next day, Voula's friend came by her home to check on her. As she left, she jokingly quipped, "Don't worry, you're just losing your mind."

With those words, Voula's air hunger returned, another panic attack struck. After that, she couldn't leave the house, couldn't drive, couldn't go to class. Her husband's impatient response was, "Shake it off!" Voula's doctor prescribed the anti-anxiety medication, sertraline, but she couldn't bring herself to take it.

Voula's crippling anxiety lasted for two years. She found help with a psychologist who acted as her anxiety coach. He taught her that anxiety is a real medical issue. The strategies that helped Voula re-enter her life included:

1. Cognitive behavioral therapy–fixing bad thinking habits

2. Diaphragmatic breathing

3. Awareness and presence training

4. Journaling

5. Gentle desensitization

Today, Voula is a college professor teaching communication and public speaking. In her class, she includes information on mindfulness and diaphragmatic breathing. These strategies come in handy when talking in front of a group of people!

Voula has come a long way. During a recent flight, as she sat in her seat, she felt the plane start to close in on her. The feeling of suffocation started. She scooted to the side as a fellow passenger went to grab something from the overhead compartment. She started to take deep breaths as she considered, "What is the worst thing that could happen to me?" As she pondered, Voula felt a sharp pain on her head and shoulder.

The man's suitcase had fallen on her head. She hadn't thought of that! Her panic waned. She smiled as she lifted the suitcase off of her, "There's no sense in worrying about what I can't control."

CHAPTER 21

Stress, anxiety and panic attacks

THE HALLMARKS OF AN ANXIETY disorder are excessive, uncontrollable worry most of the time. Worried thoughts are difficult to control and preoccupy your day. For example, you drop your son off at daycare but then you worry for hours if he is ok. You can't concentrate or get your tasks done, for hours. Anxiety makes you feel restless, on edge, and irritable. Small, everyday stressors like someone cutting you off in traffic or a snarky email spike your adrenaline levels, making you irritable for hours. Anxiety disorders manifest with physical symptoms too, through the mind-body connection.

Panic attacks are a type of anxiety disorder. The attacks represent a surge of anxiety accompanied by intense physical discomfort. They appear in a variety of ways, such as chest pain or trouble breathing. Voula experienced shortness of breath, like she was suffocating. Others experience chest pain and heart palpitations and some feel dizzy and disoriented. I experienced stomach pain with vomiting. Panic attack symptoms can last anywhere from ten minutes to hours. The discomfort is so intense, you feel like you are dying.

Panic attacks are a common reason for emergency room visits because they mimic life-threatening conditions. Chest pain like a heart attack, trouble breathing like a blood clot in the lung, or stomach pain like a bleeding ulcer. The symptoms are varied, yet they reflect the same underlying condition.

Voula struggled with panic attacks. The attacks started after she experienced a traumatic event as a child, when she witnessed a man die before her. Surviving two terrifying earthquakes cemented the disorder in her nervous system. Later as an adult, the attacks returned, provoked during times of high stress. Panic attacks are a common, stress-related disorder.

Mindfulness calms the nervous system

Since panic attacks are a stress-related disorder, their management requires consideration of stress's role in their treatment. If stress underlies the panic disorder, the attacks will continue to worsen in frequency and severity until addressed. I can vouch for that! Your body sends small signals at first, which get louder and louder if you do not listen. Until they can no longer be ignored. You wind up laid out on an emergency room stretcher, fearing you are dying like Bryan, Olivia, Voula, and I.

Mindfulness practice halts your body's stress response by calming the nervous system, which also reduces anxiety. The stress response activates the fight-or-flight response (sympathetic nervous system). Mindfulness switches the body to the rest and digest mode (parasympathetic nervous system). A recent study found it can be as helpful as medications for initial treatment of anxiety.[27]

Voula found mindfulness practice and deep breathing helpful to calm rising anxiety and halt a panic attack. She worked on self-awareness and understanding her mind-body connection. She became attuned to her anxiety ramping up and could take action before it grew out of control. She learned when her heart rate sped up and hot flashes pulsated on her neck, that air hunger was soon to follow. She used deep breathing to subdue her nervous system. This returned Voula's sense of control over her body and lowered her anxiety about her anxiety.

Diaphragmatic breathing is a form of slow, deep breathing that turns off the stress response. Deep breathing calms the nervous system, telling the brain everything is "ok," no need to prepare to fight a bear. And, it is easy to do.

Diaphragmatic breathing calms the stress response

The diaphragm is a dome-shaped muscle that helps you breathe in and out. This muscle sits below the lungs and separates your chest from your abdomen. When you breathe in, the diaphragm contracts, flattens, and moves down toward your abdomen. This movement allows your chest to get bigger and pull in air. When you breathe out, your diaphragm relaxes and moves back up as your lungs push the air out. Diaphragmatic breathing uses your lungs to their full capacity and contributes to a more relaxed state.

---

[27] Elizabeth A. Hoge et al., "Mindfulness-Based Stress Reduction vs Escitalopram for the Treatment of Adults With Anxiety Disorders: A Randomized Clinical Trial," JAMA Psychiatry 80, no. 1 (2023): 13-21. https://doi.org/10.1001/jamapsychiatry.2022.3679.

DIAPHRAGMATIC BREATHING

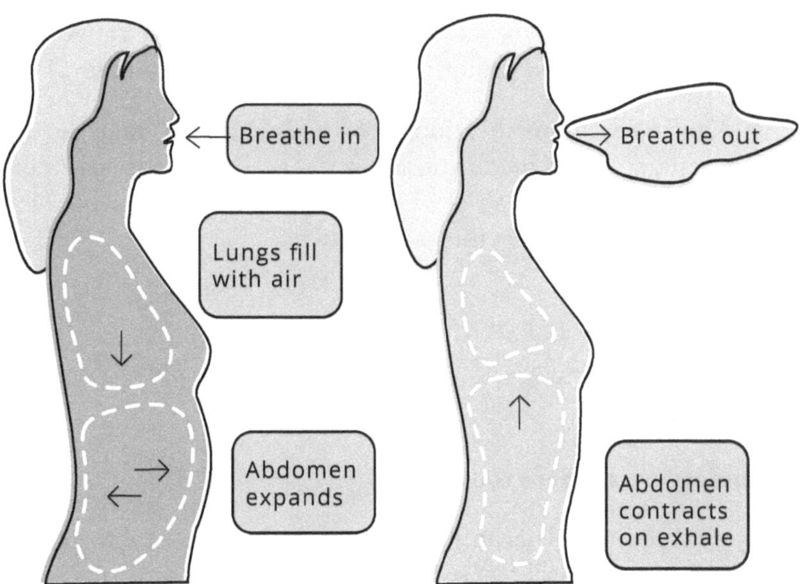

It's simple:

1. Find a comfortable place to sit or lay down.

2. Place one hand on your belly, just below your rib cage.

3. Take a slow, deep breath in through your nose over four seconds. Feel your lower belly expand as you inhale.

4. Exhale through your mouth over six seconds and feel your belly retract.

That's it! Your brain now knows everything is ok.

Start with a couple of minutes of deep breathing and expand from there. Work up to five or ten minutes. Find what works best for you.

A note on medications

When anxiety or panic disorders are severe, mindfulness and diaphragmatic breathing may not be enough. When the nervous system is firing out of control, medications are a helpful option.

You might benefit from one of the safe and effective medications that decrease anxiety and panic attacks.

- The medication group—called the SSRIs (selective serotonin reuptake inhibitors)—are effective at reducing anxiety levels. Examples include sertraline and citalopram. Although they are called "antidepressants," these medications reduce anxiety when taken in the lower dose range. There are other anxiety medication groups; SSRIs are just one example.

- Stronger anti-anxiety medications,"benzodiazepines", include diazepam and clonazepam. These medications are reserved for severe cases or to stop a panic attack. They carry a risk of addiction so they are reserved for severe cases. That said, sometimes they are needed.

> **" PART OF MANAGING ANXIETY IS
> UNDERSTANDING HOW IT FEELS IN YOU. "**

GAD-7: Anxiety awareness tool

Does axiety make you feel irritable? Does it make your stomach hurt? The Generalized Anxiety Disorder—GAD-7 is a clinical measure that helps build awareness of your anxiety levels. This tool asks how often you feel on edge, have uncontrollable worry, and other signs of anxiety.

For each of the seven statements on the GAD-7, you assess your levels, according to the criteria, ranging from "Not at all" to "Nearly every day". The maximum score is 21. A score of 10 or higher suggests moderate anxiety symptoms. A score of 15 or more indicates severe anxiety.

While the GAD-7 is useful, it doesn't ask about the physical symptoms anxiety causes, such as headaches, stomach pain, or dizziness. The PHQ-15 is a better tool to look at physical symptoms. Nonetheless, the GAD-7 is a start to building awareness of the signs of anxiety in yourself.

Simply recognizing that your symptoms are from anxiety, helps lower anxiety.

GAD-7

Over the <u>last 2 weeks</u>, how often have you been bothered by the following problems? *(Use "✔" to indicate your answer)*	Not at all	Several days	More than half the days	Nearly every day
1. Feeling nervous, anxious or on edge	0	1	2	3
2. Not being able to stop or control worrying	0	1	2	3
3. Worrying too much about different things	0	1	2	3
4. Trouble relaxing	0	1	2	3
5. Being so restless that it is hard to sit still	0	1	2	3
6. Becoming easily annoyed or irritable	0	1	2	3
7. Feeling afraid as if something awful might happen	0	1	2	3

(For office coding: Total Score T____ = ____ + ____ + ____)

Developed by Drs. Robert L. Spitzer, Janet B.W. Williams, Kurt Kroenke and colleagues, with an educational grant from Pfizer Inc. No permission required to reproduce, translate, display or distribute.

BOTTOM LINE

Anxiety disorders bring about uncontrollable worry and persistent fear of bad things occurring. They are associated with an amped up nervous system that makes you feel irritable and on edge. Anxiety and panic attacks can both appear with physical symptoms, such as chest pain, trouble breathing, abdominal pain, headaches, or dizziness.

The GAD-7 is an anxiety awareness tool to help connect you to the signs of anxiety in yourself. The practice of mindfulness and diaphragmatic breathing calm the nervous system. If these strategies are not enough, there are safe and effective medications available.

CHAPTER 22

Correcting cognitive distortions...stay with me, this is interesting

FRIEND: "LISA, I LOVE THAT OUTFIT."

Lisa: *"The outfit would look better if I lost ten pounds, I am so overweight."*

Manager: "Lisa, your work on that project was brilliant!"

Lisa: *"Well, I had help."*

Co-worker: "Lisa, you are so smart."

Lisa: *"No, I just spend a lot of time reading."*

Friend: "Lisa, you are so kind. How do you find the time to do all that volunteer work?"

Lisa: *"Mother Theresa did more..."*

Lisa sounds humble, right? And that might be exactly what her friends, co-workers, and manager believe.

Humility might not be a positive attribute. It could be a sign of unhealthy thinking.

Lisa's comments reflect cognitive distortions. Cognitive distortions are bad thinking habits. Thinking in a way that not only distorts reality, but also makes you feel bad. For example, Lisa picks out a negative aspect in each interaction, dismissing the positive. Her thoughts are turning outward compliments into inward insults. Lisa shows the cognitive distortion of mental filtering; she dwells on the bad and ignores the good. Does this sound familiar?

The process of working on healthy thought patterns and reducing cognitive distortions is called cognitive behavioral therapy (CBT), developed by psychiatrist Aaron Beck in the 1960s.

> " CBT WORKS ON IMPROVING AWARENESS THAT OUR THOUGHTS AND PERCEPTIONS OF A SITUATION DON'T NECESSARILY REFLECT THE ACTUAL REALITY OF IT. "

Especially if we are taking a biased, negative perspective about it, like Lisa.

Turn off the negative thinking

Reducing cognitive distortions reduces negative thoughts, which reduces negative emotions. This, in turn, reduces the stress response and calms the nervous system. Revered psychiatrists Aaron Beck and David Burns introduced the following categories of cognitive distortions:

1. All-or-nothing thinking—With this type of distortion, you think about yourself or the world in absolute, black-or-white terms. You evaluate your personal qualities in extreme ways as either incredible or horrible. For example, if a work project turns out poorly, you think you are terrible at your job. If another project goes well, you think you are amazing. You are either really good or really bad, with no in-between. In reality, most of the time, situations are somewhere in the middle, with shades of gray. Most likely, you are not fluctuating from zero percent to one hundred percent performance. Yet, holding onto the thought that you are horrible generates negative emotions like sadness and shame. But, the thought is not accurate. The thought is not reality. The thought is a distortion.

I caught myself using this distortion during the clinic. I fluctuated between "I am pretty good at patient care" to "I am horrible at patient care." In reality, I am somewhere in the middle. I am not the worst or the best.

Try it: Invest a few hours and monitor your thoughts for extreme, black-or-white thinking. If you catch yourself in an extreme thought, pause, then take a minute to reframe your thought to one less extreme and closer to reality.

2. Overgeneralization—With overgeneralization, you make a broad conclusion about yourself based on a single event. You take one negative event and generalize it to a never ending pattern of defeat. The keywords to watch out for are talking to yourself in "always" and "never" terms. For example, I have a doctor friend, Alyssa, who is kind, responsible, and considered attractive. In medical school, the guys literally tripped over each other trying to talk to her. Every day, for about a year. I was in my usual role as the cute friend of the really hot girl. The point being, there were always interested parties for Alyssa.

Anyway, when a long-term relationship ended, she told me she was unlovable. She would never find a partner. Now, I know this person. I can say she is absolutely lovable. Her generalization from her last relationship ending to the thought she was "unlovable" is a distortion of reality. In reality, she was loved. In reality, a relationship breaking up does not mean a person is unlovable. It more likely signifies the two people are different or incompatible or one hundred other things. The facts do not support such a harsh, extreme conclusion.

Alyssa's thought about being unlovable was clearly distorted, but her heart believed it. She burst into tears as she proclaimed she was unlovable. Thoughts are powerful.

Try it: Focus on catching yourself making "always" or "never" statements. If you make one, take a few moments to correct the thought using objective information. How do you feel after you've made this adjustment?

3. Mental filter—With a mental filter, you dwell on the negative and ignore the positives. If mental filtering were a sport, I would be an elite athlete. A medal contender. This is the process of picking out the negative details in any situation and dwelling on them, while ignoring or discounting the positive information.

For example, my boss told me I did an amazing job on my spinal injection presentation, that I knocked it out of the park. I dismissed the compliment. Instead,

I thought to myself, "Well, it was only good because I spent ten hours on it. Everyone else probably completed their presentations in five hours. Probably." My thoughts completely discounted the positives. I had no idea how much time the other doctors had spent. I not only dismissed the positive comment, I created a negative thought from it. I turned the positive comment into an insult in my head. That is an impressive cognitive distortion.

A Gratitude Journal helped me neutralize my negative mental filter. My propensity to discount the positives. Each night before bed, I wrote down three positive events about my day. Anything counted, big or small. A great cup of coffee. An enjoyable conversation with the barista who made my coffee. The sun shining. Living in a place where the sun shines. Keeping a Gratitude Journal tuned my brain to the positive. I started to instinctively see more positives in my day. The negative patterns weakened. So simple, but so effective.

Try it: Start a Gratitude Journal. Commit to writing down at least three positive events from your day or three things you're grateful for. Remember, it doesn't matter how small or simple an event was. If something has added to the quality of your day, write it down! Also, get in the habit of rereading your entries.

4. Jumping to conclusions—mind reading and fortune telling

You can make a quick assumption using one of two ways.

Mind reading—I observe this cognitive distortion causing the most chaos between people. Mind reading is when people assume they know what someone else is thinking or why someone else is doing something. Then, they get upset over their own thoughts about the person's actions.

For example, I recently headed to the pharmacy to get a question answered. Reaching the pharmacy by phone had become impossible, so I decided to stop in. At the counter, I started asking my question.

"The prescription notification system…"

The pharmacy employee interrupted me and said "Oh, you want text alerts. I will sign you up for text alerts." She dutifully started signing me up.

"Well, no, that was not my question." I started again, "The prescription notification system…"

Again, she interrupted and said, "There is nothing ready for you."

"Well, no, I am not here for a prescription." I tried again, "The prescription notification system…."

The employee again interrupted me. "What is your date of birth?"

For whatever reason, she was unable to listen to my entire sentence to hear my actual request: "The prescription notification system does not tell me when a prescription cannot be filled. I am submitting prescriptions, but they are not being filled."

When I realized this person was not going to hear me out, I said, "Thank you," and left the pharmacy. As I walked outside, my phone beeped. I looked down. I was now signed up for text alerts from the pharmacy.

With mind reading, the person assumes they know what's in your head. They think they know what you are going to say. Except, they don't. They have no insight that their perspective does not reflect your reality.

Miscommunication as a result of mind reading runs rampant on social media. People interpret a post through the narrow lens of their world, past experiences, and culture. Since they do not understand the lens and context of the person posting, they misunderstand the intended meaning. They have negative thoughts, which then trigger negative emotions, like anger or outrage. These people respond with angry or mean comments. The thing is, it is their own perceptions that are sparking these emotions, not the reality.

On social media, there are no facial expressions or voice intonations to clarify the intent of a post or comment. There is limited context. An emoji might help but that is also left up to interpretation. Malice is too often assumed. Apology posts follow. Social media is a cognitive distortion superfest!

Dr. Burns, in his book *Feeling Great*, discusses how to minimize mind reading. First, you need to develop awareness that you are doing it. That's a big step right there. We're so often unaware of our behaviors.

Once you develop awareness, you can focus on asking people what they are thinking and feeling, rather than guessing. And, in turn, sharing how you think and feel since others cannot know otherwise.

Try it: Take a few hours each day and work on catching yourself mind reading when you're interacting with others. Pay attention to the voice in your head. If you catch yourself mind reading, pause, and allow them to finish the sentence. You can ask clarifying questions afterwards.

For example, the pharmacy worker from my example was trying to read my mind, quite unsuccessfully. She should have paused and clarified, "Do you want to be signed up for text alerts?" I would have said, "No, I do not want to be signed up for text alerts. I want to understand why I can't get my prescriptions." Even better, she could have let me complete my sentence.

Fortune telling—Fortune telling is another form of jumping to conclusions. With this distortion, you predict the worst case scenario will happen without supporting evidence. For example, your partner is away for the day on a business trip. You fear he is at a club with his colleagues. And he is cheating on you. Then you're anxious that your relationship is over. You believe this negative thought even though your partner has never cheated or shown signs of cheating in the past. There is no evidence supporting these worries and fears.

Try it: If you are worried something terrible is going to happen, pause, and write down your fears. Next to your fears, write down the evidence or likelihood of the feared outcome happening. If there is no evidence for your feared outcome, you have caught yourself fortune telling.

5. Magnification and minimization—When you magnify the negative and minimize the positive, exaggerating the reality, you're engaging in the cognitive distortion of magnification and minimization. For instance, from a personal standpoint, you magnify your flaws, but minimize your strengths. You maximize your intellectual shortcomings, while you minimize your positive traits, like being well-liked, caring, and generous. If you are emphasizing your flaws and dismissing your strengths, you lower your value, chipping away at your self-worth.

Try it: One way to neutralize magnification and minimization is to challenge your negative thought by writing down the objective facts. Do the facts support the thought? The more objective the approach, the closer to reality a thought becomes.

6. Emotional reasoning—This distortion uses your feelings and emotions to draw conclusions. For example, you feel bad at your job so you conclude that you ARE bad at your job. You feel worthless, so you must BE worthless. The problem with this type of thinking is that how you feel in the moment is not an accurate measurement from which to make a broad—and potentially damaging—determination.

As Dr. Burns wrote, just because you feel something strongly doesn't make it true. Emotions result from our thoughts and our thoughts are often distorted. Feelings don't represent reality. When you feel something strongly, it's natural to conclude that it must be true. But it's not. You need to recognize when a negative thought is actually a distortion.

Try it: Challenge your emotional reasoning by going back to objective statements and facts. If you're feeling worthless, challenge the emotion. Write down three things you accomplished in the last year. Maybe it's about the work you do or about the children you care for. Maybe it is about the friend you were there for. Do the three things you wrote down support that you are worthless?

7. "Should" statements create unnecessary suffering. They reflect regret, resentment, and guilt. This type of cognitive distortion involves the critical "he/she/I should have X."—what someone should have done or should be like. Negative "should" statements are a form of non-productive judgment.

Judging others creates negative emotions, such as anger and resentment. The judgment doesn't change anyone, but the toxicity festers and eats away at you. Judging others hurts you. Instead of criticizing others, try accepting them for who they are. Letting go of judging others is freeing and brings peace.

Try it: Spend a few hours being aware of when you make negative "should" statements about yourself or others. If you catch yourself in a "should" statement, observe the feelings that resulted from your "shoulds". Did the statement intensify negative emotions? Did the statement solve anything? Awareness is the start to healing.

8. Labeling is when you call yourself a negative name, like "stupid." Labeling is an overgeneralization and triggers negative emotions. The label is unlikely to accurately reflect who you are. For example, you make a mistake and proclaim that one mistake makes you stupid. Rather than labeling yourself as stupid, bring the self-talk closer to reality, "I made a mistake, I am disappointed." A more objective thought. Labeling is an oversimplification.

Try it: Monitor your thoughts to see if you catch yourself using negative labels. When you find yourself labeling, make a clarifying thought that is objective with no label.

9. Blaming—You fault yourself or others for an error. For example, your son is hospitalized at three months old because you placed him in daycare, not understanding the risks of placing a premature newborn in daycare. Blaming does not resolve an issue, but actually prolongs its impact. After it has happened, feel your emotions, learn from the experience, and move forward.

Try it: Monitor your thoughts and see if you catch yourself blaming—yourself or others. When you find yourself blaming, correct the thought.

BOTTOM LINE

Reading through all the types of cognitive distortions might be overwhelming. I recommend starting by picking out the distortion you find yourself doing the most often. Work on that one for a week. Spend a few hours each day intentionally monitoring your thoughts to catch and correct it. With time, your mind will adapt and make fewer distortions. Healthier thought patterns will emerge. Repeat this process each week, focusing on a different distortion each time. You will find reducing distortions lowers anxiety levels and increases happiness levels.

For a more in-depth study on cognitive distortions, I recommend reading Dr. David Burns' book, *Feeling Great*. Additionally, for more guided work, psychologists are skilled in working with people to reduce cognitive distortions.

CHAPTER 23

Jenna's story: Hard-working mom goes numb from stress

JENNA WAS A 30-YEAR-OLD PATENT attorney and mom with a precious four-year-old son named Chase. Although she was married, nearly all of the childcare lay on Jenna's shoulders. Her son had big, blue eyes and an even bigger heart. Chase was on the autism spectrum. He needed extra help with talking and communicating in an understandable way. Jenna and Chase attended speech therapy a few days each week. She spent hours each week studying the developmental differences of a neurodivergent child; she felt she needed a PhD in parenting to successfully navigate the complexity.

Chase also had sensory processing differences that caused him to experience pain and become overwhelmed in areas with numerous people, loud sounds, or strong smells. His intense senses could not tolerate the smells from a restaurant, the noise of a movie theater, or the number of people at an indoor playground. In these high stimulation environments, he collapsed into a sensory meltdown. His nervous system was so overwhelmed, so overstimulated that he would scream or run around uncontrollably until he was moved to a quieter place. Meanwhile, Jenna felt the searing glares of others judging her and Chase. They assumed Chase's poor behavior stemmed from her parenting rather than a neurodivergent child trying to exist in a world that was not designed with neurodivergence in mind.

It took years before Jenna understood why Chase was so out of control in public places, yet so calm at home. Her pediatrician's office staff empathetically stated how difficult he was and complimented her for doing a good job. They didn't seem to understand or pick up on the sensory processing issues. They focused on Chase's asthma. His asthma was well-controlled.

At home, in a quiet environment, Chase was the most loving soul. He had an interesting perspective on the world, seeing things Jenna didn't. He saw things the world didn't. The little boy noticed details. He noticed people. Everything Jenna thought she knew about autism was wrong. Chase's brain was wired differently but in the most fascinating ways. If only the glaring, judgmental observers could see this, too. If they could just see the gifts that neurodivergence brings, instead of just the disability. This disconnect from the world around her was stressful.

Jenna worked as a patent attorney in Seattle, and she was a smart one. She enjoyed working with aspiring innovators, writing up their latest ideas for patent submissions. She yawned at all the big corporate patents she churned out but felt purpose when drafting a patent for a local inventor. But she felt increasingly deficient in her ability to do good legal work and be a good mom to Chase.

Going numb

When I met Jenna, she was calm and composed but looked somber. With worried eyes, she explained that the right side of her body had started going numb for a few hours at a time. The numbness had started a few months earlier and had increased in frequency. Now, the numbness in her right arm and leg occurred weekly and remained longer. Jenna was concerned that she might have developed a serious neurologic disorder, like multiple sclerosis (MS).

Seattle has a high rate of MS. We blame the statistic on the lack of sun, given the higher rates of MS in the North. Well…and genetics. Genetics always contributes something.

The numbness on Jenna's right side did not follow the pattern of the nerves in the body. Usually, numbness appears in the region of the damaged nerves. That said, the body doesn't always adhere to the neurology textbook when developing disease, so we pursued a thorough evaluation. Testing returned negative for a traditional type of neurologic disorder, such as multiple sclerosis or brain tumor.

Let me clarify. Jenna's test results were negative for a medical disorder with a visible area of damage that I could point to and explain her symptoms. The negative workup did not mean Jenna was ok.

Her symptoms indicated a serious problem. Her body was beyond stressed, at its breaking point, and screaming for help. In her case, long-standing overwhelming stress triggered her neurologic symptoms. She was suffering from a stress-related disorder called functional neurologic disorder (FND or conversion disorder). With FND, the person develops motor or sensory deficits, such as weakness or numbness, with no neurologic explanation. There is not a visible tumor or stroke. The problem cannot be visualized by medical tests. Frequently, conversion is precipitated by an acute stressor, trauma, or adverse life event. The psychological distress that accompanies FND results in physical symptoms that are not consciously controlled by the person. They are not faking; they feel one side is numb or weak.

Mind-body disorder

How psychological stress results in physical symptoms is poorly understood. The lack of understanding is perhaps why there is so much stigma and negative judgment around it. When FND develops in a person, providers have a hard time explaining the reason. From conversations with my provider friends and patients, medical professionals get uncomfortable trying to communicate that a condition is a "mind-body" disorder. The provider tenses up and has trouble finding the words to explain what is occurring. They fear the patient will take the information the wrong way and get angry. So, they refer the patient to a psychologist. The lack of explanation with a psychology referral does not go over well. People end up feeling like no one believes them. It's a hurtful dismissal. I can confirm, patients do take an unexplained psychology referral the wrong way!

Advances in functional imaging have begun to provide clues to how psychological stress results in physical symptoms. Functional imaging shows what areas of the brain are active during certain tasks, such as picking up an object or during experiences, such as feeling back pain or leg numbness. Research has revealed there is a change in the brain's processing of information in people with a conversion disorder. Areas of the brain that are activated by emotional stress lead to reduced sensory or motor processing.[28] For Jenna, overwhelming stress caused the nerves to be unable to process sensory information on one side, thus the numbness.

Another example is when strength (motor processing) is affected by a mind-body disorder. In the inpatient rehabilitation unit, patients who experienced strokes, brain injuries, and spinal cord injuries undergo an intensive program of rehabilitation to maximize recovery. A few times per year, a patient with FND was admitted for stroke-like symptoms. They presented with weakness on one side, just like a stroke. They could not move their arm or leg, but no stroke could be seen on imaging. They could not lift their arm if you asked them. But,

---

[28] Samuel B. Harvey, Biba R. Stanton, and Anthony S. David, "Conversion Disorder: Towards a Neurobiological Understanding," Neuropsychiatric Disease and Treatment 2, no. 1 (2006): 13-20.

if you paid close attention, you could catch them performing automatic movements, like scratching using the arm they could not consciously move. Automatic movements are preserved in FND.

Awareness Journal

Let's go back to Jenna. Her long-standing, overwhelming stress triggered numbness. So, what now? There was no life stress dial we could just turn down. We first needed to build awareness of her symptom triggers.

I recommended Jenna keep an Awareness Journal to track when the numbness episodes occurred to build mind-body awareness. She wrote down where she felt numbness, what she was doing, and how she was feeling when it occurred. After a few weeks, we looked for patterns. Did the numbness follow a twelve-hour workday? Sleep deprivation days? Sick child days? Days or weeks with all three?

The Awareness Journal revealed a pattern. The numbness occurred during time spans, weeks at a time, when she was on a tight work deadline and Chase was having frequent meltdowns. Of note, an autistic or neurodivergent meltdown is not your typical tantrum. The episodes can last for hours as their little bodies struggle to self-regulate.

Journaling also uncovered other insights. Her writings exposed that Jenna felt she was always failing as a mother or as an attorney or both. When she did her work well, she didn't feel she was meeting Chase's needs. When she met Chase's needs, her work suffered. She felt bad at everything. And that made her feel worse. Feeling like a bad mother and a bad attorney was a stressful combination for Jenna.

Tough talk

Jenna and I had a difficult conversation as I explained that the level of stress she was under was breaking her body down. The demands had provoked a stress-related disorder. If her stress level was not lowered, her condition would get worse. The conversation was tough because I was painfully aware of how unrealistic it is to tell a working mother to just "reduce stress." No less, a working mother with a special needs child. Like she was working herself sick by choice. Like she wouldn't get more help if she could. Like she wouldn't secure more resources for Chase if available.

That said, I found it helpful to give people permission to take care of themselves. Pointing out their body was physically breaking down helped. Clarifying they were not weak helped. Reassuring them they were not alone helped.

Jenna and I discussed what taking care of herself would look like. We created a specific plan. What needed to happen to improve the situation? For Jenna, she needed to reduce the total number of weekly demands between work and parenting. She reduced her work hours from full-time to three-quarters time. No more taking on additional work projects.

Then, she adjusted her "mom schedule". Normally, each week Chase attended speech therapy to help with his communication and occupational therapy to work on sensory differences. Reluctantly, but realistically, Jenna reduced the number of therapy visits they attended each week. Occasionally, they even took a two-week "therapy break"—a special needs vacation to just be present. Jenna needed a schedule she could sustain over the long term.

The awareness builds

While making these changes, Jenna continued to keep an Awareness Journal to track her symptoms. This activity strengthened her mind-body connection. She noticed how, as the feeling of being overwhelmed grew, her right arm and then her leg would start to tingle. Just making the connection that her right side was going numb due to being overwhelmed helped her pause and recalibrate demand levels. Developing awareness of what the numbness represented decreased it. Jenna made the mind-body connection; numbness was a physical signal to slow down and take care of herself.

Jenna let go of striving to be the absolute perfect parent and the absolute perfect career woman at the absolute same time. Over the next six months, Jenna's symptoms improved. The numbness episodes decreased in frequency from weekly to every few months. When the numbness returned, it was a signal she needed to pull back from her "to-do" list and prioritize her health.

For Jenna, building awareness and reducing her stress level were the key factors for healing. No other medications or interventions were needed. Her stress response had remained in the "on" position for too long. She worked a demanding job during the day and cared for her special needs son at night, enduring too many hard days over far too many years. She had no time for rest or recovery. Long-term, overwhelming stress provoked her medical disorder. And the condition improved when she made a conscious effort to reduce the demands on herself.

BOTTOM LINE

Jenna became overwhelmed by all the roles she fulfilled, between her career as a lawyer and parenting a special needs child. Pulled in two different directions every day for years, Jenna felt like she was being ripped in two. She developed a stress-related disorder that resulted in the right side of her body going numb. The numbness was a physical sign that she needed to reduce demands. Starting an Awareness Journal brought Jenna in touch with triggers and enabled her to make the mind-body connection. Over time, awareness of how stress affected her physically grew. She was empowered to set boundaries to maintain her health.

CHAPTER 24

Burnout: Stress rewires the brain... and not in a good way

SINCE YOU'RE READING *SUNBREAK,* YOU'RE probably all too familiar with burnout. You feel physically and emotionally exhausted. Stress has drained all the energy and motivation. What's really going on when you feel this way?

High stress levels not only trigger medical conditions, they change how your brain works. High levels of uncontrollable work stress impair prefrontal cortex (PFC) function.[29] I call the PFC the "diplomatic lobe" of your brain. This area helps you regulate your thoughts, actions, and emotions. And it helps with insight, reasoning, and decision-making.

The prefrontal cortex keeps you civil in a conflict. For example, this part of the brain prevents you from punching a stranger in the face when they are mean to your child. It stops you from screaming at your boss who is unreasonable. That is, the prefrontal cortex can do this when it's functioning well. Uncontrollable stress or overload weakens PFC functioning. Fatigue and sleep deprivation, common with overload, also weaken the PFC. When the PFC can't perform, you become short-tempered and make poor decisions.

While high stress inhibits the diplomatic lobe, it strengthens the more primitive, reflexive brain areas, like the amygdala and brainstem. With the onslaught of stress, the parts of the brain that allow higher-order thinking and self-regulation are weakened, while survival behaviors and reflexive responses are strengthened. Essentially, it's the exact opposite of what you want going on during the work day.

---

[29] Amy FT Arnsten, "Stress Weakens Prefrontal Networks: Molecular Insults to Higher Cognition," Nature Neuroscience 18, no. 10 (October 2015): 1376-1385.

YOUR BRAIN UNDER STRESS

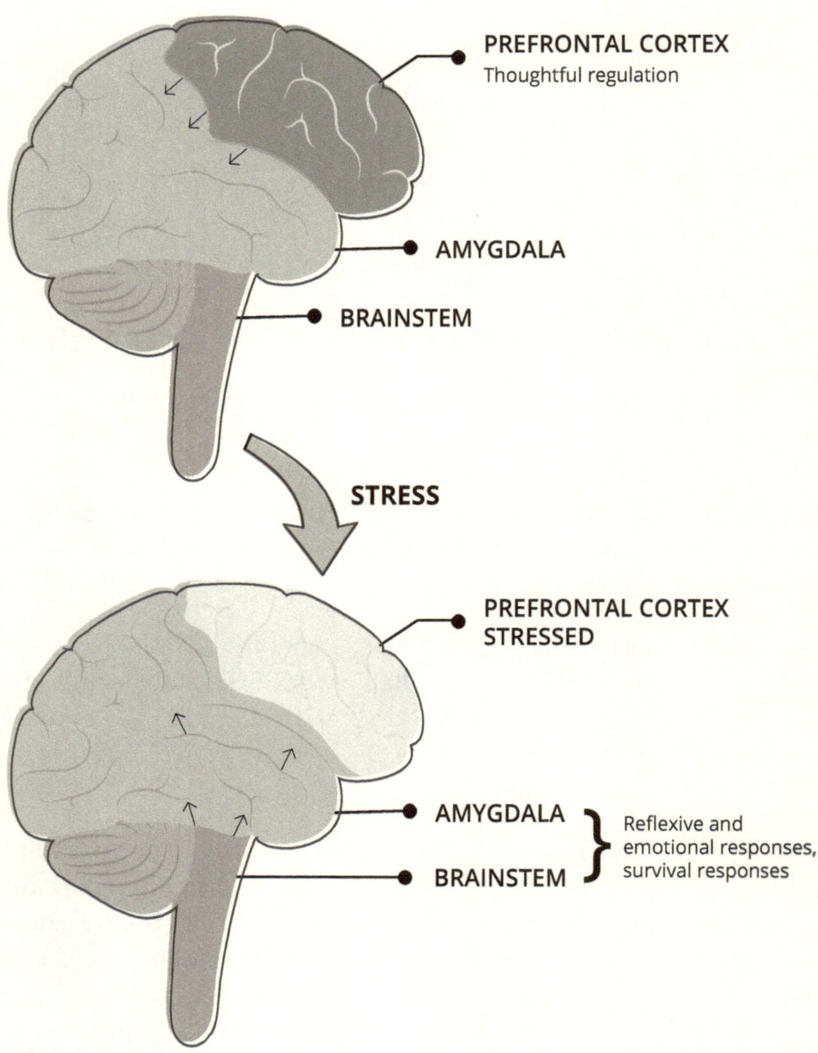

These changes don't occur if the stress is controllable. If you feel confident you can handle a situation and sufficient resources are at hand, the PFC continues to function. And, prefrontal connections return to normal during sustained periods of non-stress. That means you can heal the damage!

The smoke signals of burnout

The changes to the diplomatic lobe and amygdala coincide with the behaviors seen with professional burnout—a state of complete mental exhaustion caused by the heavy demands of work life. It stems from long-standing, unmanageable work stress combined with high ideals. Perfectionists are particularly at risk, because they don't give their minds and bodies a break!

Three main characteristics of burnout are: emotional exhaustion, detachment and reduced work effectiveness or sense of accomplishment.[30]

1. Extreme emotional exhaustion. This is not simply an exhausting day, but years of beyond exhausting days. Years of feeling overworked, overextended, and having nothing left to give. This was Jenna's emotional state that led to her stress-related disorder.

2. Detachment. A distance and indifference grows between you and the work. Work that once had meaning and purpose no longer does. For example, a former colleague of mine was working at a health insurance agency. Lauren went from feeling she was helping people to feeling that her work made no difference. In the past, she had enjoyed the gratification gained from helping people access medical care. As she developed burnout, she no longer believed her efforts mattered.

3. Reduced work effectiveness and sense of accomplishment. Reduced work effectiveness means you're not doing the job to your standard. You feel incompetent or inefficient. For example, Jenna no longer felt she was doing acceptable work. She felt rushed. She struggled to meet deadlines. A 90 percent effort did not feel adequate; too much was at stake for her clients. Torn between work and home responsibilities, Jenna's burnout was all-encompassing.

A concept you're familiar with at this point, awareness, is the first step to managing burnout. The insidious onset of burnout can be hard to detect. It's difficult to see in yourself—to see what's happening when you're stuck in the murkiness of it all. Unending exhaustion, growing indifference, and feeling bad about your job are signs to look for. With awareness, you can step back, get a better view, and take the action needed for a healthy change. Hopefully, you do this before a stress-related medical condition develops.

Burnout Management 101

Get ready. Now comes the hard part: setting reasonable boundaries. This is especially tough when a power imbalance exists between you and the boundary that needs to be set. Or, the work environment is predatory. Medical residency is predatory by design. You are $200,000 in debt and must complete your resi-

---

[30] Brian E. Lacy and Johanna L. Chan, "Physician Burnout: The Hidden Health Care Crisis," Clinical Gastroenterology and Hepatology 16, no. 3 (March 2018): 311–17.

dency to graduate and work as a physician.

I recall, during my year in internal medicine, being taught that I did not have boundaries. There was no such thing as saying "no." Restrictions on sleeping, eating, and using the bathroom were standard. I suppose this is where the need for the eighty-hour work week rule emanated from. In 2003, the Council for Graduate Medical Education implemented rules limiting doctors in their residencies to working a maximum of eighty hours per week. This rule was controversial at the time; some felt eighty hours was too restrictive. True, the hours add up quickly when you have multiple thirty-six-hour shifts per week.

I vividly remember during my first year of residency being punished by my senior resident for not responding to a page in less than sixty seconds. The page was for a non-urgent matter at two in the morning and I was using the restroom. There was a different system in place for urgent matters. I don't recall my punishment, but it had to do with more sleep deprivation. That same year, in December, as the holidays approached, a different senior resident told us if we got sick and called out, we'd better not come back unless we had a hospital discharge summary to prove we had been sick. He warned unless we were sick enough to be admitted to the hospital, we couldn't call in sick for work. Being the overly compliant people pleaser I was, I am sure I worked for three weeks in a hospital with a punishing case of bronchitis.

Setting boundaries is a hard concept to understand if you are not used to having basic rights, like eating, sleeping, or being sick. In retrospect, a training program on how to deal with power-hungry senior residents would have been helpful! I did not have awareness they were over-stepping boundaries, nor did I understand my rights under their direction.

Recognizing when work demands have become unreasonable is difficult for those with people-pleasing tendencies (like me). We have a natural tendency to accommodate everyone else's needs, even if they severely undermine our own. As opposed to those with more self-directed personalities, those who are driven more by their individual choices rather than what makes those around them happy. It's not an all-or-nothing personality. You can learn to explore, set, and maintain boundaries.

How to say "no" the right way

Do you find it hard to say "no" to people? Here are tips to set boundaries in a kind, direct, and clear manner.

- Be straightforward and direct. Say "no" or "I can't" as opposed to "I don't think so" or "maybe" which leaves your answer open to negotiation. Make your answer clear.

- Briefly explain yourself, respectfully, in one to two sentences. "I just took on a major project with a tight deadline" or "My schedule is full." A brief explanation provides context to why you are saying no. Your decision should be understood and respected.

- Offer an alternative option, if it applies. "Here are some resources and people that may be able to help." Pointing them in the right direction is appreciated.

Here are a few scripts.

"No, I won't be able to fit that into my schedule this week."

"I can't assist, but here are a few resources you may find helpful."

"No, I need to prioritize a, b, and c."

"That sounds fun, but my schedule is full at the moment."

"I can't commit time right now."

Strike out the stressor

Another strategy to reduce burnout is increasing your control over the stressor. When you feel confident about a situation and have adequate resources to deal with the burden, it's not as stressful. For example, let's say I am a resident working in the ICU for the first time. I have three critically ill patients, one with a stomach bleed, one in a diabetic coma, and one in heart failure. My senior resident brushes me off and won't help. The nurse for these patients is brand new with no experience. I feel on my own with critical stakes; these patients are at high risk of death. Super stressful!

Now let's take the same situation, first week in the ICU with three critically ill patients, but change the resources. My senior resident is supportive and is ready and available for questions. The nurse has 30 years of experience in the ICU and knows what to do before I write the order. The situation is still stressful, but I feel supported and confident the patients will have a positive outcome. You can't always control the resources available to you, but developing an awareness of the resources you need and asking for them is the first step in managing a stressful environment.

Regaining control can take on multiple forms from resource management, to work schedule changes, to larger changes involving career shaping. Careers can look a variety of ways. A doctor can do patient care. From there, she chooses to do outpatient clinic or hospital care. Another route, or shape, a doctor can do non-clinical care. She can work in hospital administration or work in health-care policy. Alternatively, she could focus on research within an academic hospital or biotechnology company.

We saw Jenna, Bryan, and Melissa mold their careers after developing a stress-related disorder:

Jenna's solution was straightforward. A valued employee, she reduced her hours per week and reduced her parenting commitments per week.

Bryan's fix was more involved. He hired two employees and delegated pieces of the work to them. A careful balance of adding help without eroding the slim profit margins of the business.

Melissa did not see a modifiable solution to her make-up business and closed it. With recovery, she re-entered the workforce initially as an employee in a different field, house painting. With time, she gained independence and her own projects. The level of control, time demands, and profit margins were a good fit.

Try it. A helpful exercise to help with career-shaping involves understanding what work activities energize and excite you, versus what drains you.

Journal your answers to these two questions:

1. What work activities drain your energy?

2. What work activities energize you?

This exercise provides perspective on the job tasks that will move you toward health. Based on the two lists, can your current situation be modified? Is there a way to do it differently? Look at your processes, the people you work with, the timelines, and the environment where you work. What can be amended? Or is it better to reshape what work looks like with a new opportunity?

Another piece to reducing burnout is increasing your level of self-care, the elusive "me" time. The most basic self-care needs include adequate sleep, good nutrition, regular exercise, and social connection with supportive friends and family. That's the starting point. From there, add in activities that make you happy. Schedule time for them. Make self-care a priority.

FOLLOW YOUR ENERGY. IT WILL LEAD YOU
TO A HAPPY, HEALTHY PATH.

BOTTOM LINE

Stress sucks the motivation and fun out of life. It also shifts your brain from human to reptilian functioning, dominated by primitive drives and reflexes, as opposed to thoughtful responsiveness. Signs of impending burnout include emotional exhaustion, indifference, and reduced work effectiveness. Managing burnout boils down to developing awareness that it's sneaking in, setting boundaries, and regaining control with career or life redesign.

CHAPTER 25

The troublemakers: Stirring up chronic inflammation

STRESS HAS ANOTHER DIRTY SECRET: It contributes to chronic low-grade inflammation. Acute inflammation occurs after an injury or infection and it helps the body heal. With chronic inflammation, the immune cells stay active, which is harmful to the body. Like an unwanted house guest who won't leave and keeps going through your things, messing everything up. The hormones and other messengers released during the stress response switch on this inflammatory, trouble-making response.[31]

Chronic inflammation—or the troublemakers—represents one way that stress leads to disease. They play a role in the development of pain conditions as well. The troublemakers cause low-grade inflammation, which messes up the nerves by sensitizing them. This step is followed by the development of a sensitization syndrome in a vulnerable part of the body.[32]

Stress → low-grade inflammation → sensitization of nerves → sensitization syndrome

Sensitization is driven by inflammation in the nervous system, called neuroinflammation. The troublemakers trespass. They are a bad influence on the glial cells in the nervous system. The glial cells are supporting cells for the nerves

---

[31] Yun-Zi Liu, Yun-Xia Wang, and Chun-Lei Jiang, "Inflammation: The Common Pathway of Stress-Related Diseases," Frontiers in Human Neuroscience 11 (June 2017). https://doi.org/10.3389/fnhum.2017.00316.

[32] Wen Zhou, JingWen Meng, and Ji Zhang, "Does Low Grade Systemic Inflammation Have a Role in Chronic Pain?," Frontiers in Molecular Neuroscience 14 (November 2021). https://doi.org/10.3389/fnmol.2021.785214.

that maintain a healthy environment for them. The troublemakers trick the glial cells into releasing inflammation-causing messengers. The messengers increase sensitivity of the nerves. Trouble-maker induced neuroinflammation is one driver of sensitization and chronic pain.[33]

Troublemakers mess with the whole body

Chronic inflammation has harmful effects on the entire body. For example, metabolic syndrome is a group of risk factors for cardiovascular disease—including high blood pressure, high blood sugar, obesity, and cholesterol abnormalities. The bad inflammation from the troublemakers in your body increases the risk of metabolic syndrome, heart disease, stroke, and diabetes.[34] The gang takes over the whole territory. The troublemakers—bad inflammation—thrive with chronic high stress, poor diet, obesity, and a sedentary lifestyle.

Let's take a closer look at how stress affects metabolic syndrome, the precursor to cardiovascular disease. Researchers looked at the association between the two over a fourteen-year time period. They defined work stress as work environments with high demands and low control. They found those with chronic work stress were more than twice as likely to develop metabolic syndrome. As stress levels went up, so did the risk of metabolic syndrome. These findings support an association between chronic psychosocial stress and the risk of chronic heart disease.[35]

As you can see, the troublemakers really mess things up, and stress is a factor they thrive on. Lowering inflammation levels will reduce your risk of developing heart disease, diabetes, and stroke. And, potentially, chronic pain states as well. To reduce these troublemakers, work on stress management, optimizing nutrition, maintaining a healthy weight, and regular physical activity.

Anti-inflammatory nutrition—healthy eating rebranded

Nutrition and gut health are important factors for reducing chronic inflammation. Gut health includes microbiome health. The microbiome consists of the bacteria and other microbes that live in the gastrointestinal tract. It plays a

---

[33] Ru-Rong Ji et al., "Neuroinflammation and Central Sensitization in Chronic and Widespread Pain," Anesthesiology 129, no. 2 (August 2018): 343–366. https://doi.org/10.1097/aln.0000000000002130.

[34] David Furman et al., "Chronic Inflammation in the Etiology of Disease Across the Life Span," Nature Medicine 25 (December 2019): 1822-1832.

[35] Tarani Chandola, Eric Brunner, and Michael Marmot, "Chronic Stress at Work and the Metabolic Syndrome: Prospective Study," BMJ 332 (2006): 521–525. https://doi.org/10.1136/bmj.38693.435301.80.

role in digestion and inflammation. The microbes help maintain the intestinal barrier, protect against pathogens, and aid proper immune function. The foods you eat can help or harm the microbiome.

Your eating habits can raise or lower inflammation levels. Eating whole foods, plenty of fruits and vegetables, and minimally processed foods lowers inflammation. The Mediterranean-style diet is a healthy example. This diet is rich in fish, fruits, nuts and seeds, olive oil, vegetables, and whole grains. Meanwhile, it is low in red meats, refined grains, saturated fats, and sugars. The Mediterranean diet is linked with lower inflammation levels and lower risk of chronic disease. On the other hand, a diet low in fruits and vegetables and high in processed foods increases inflammation levels. It also alters the gut microbiome in a negative way. I have been eating an anti-inflammatory diet for the past five years. My skin looks younger and brighter. I have more energy too.

Physical activity

Regular physical activity lowers inflammation levels. The primary goal of exercise is to find what works for your body, your energy level, and your schedule. You don't have to get up at five a.m. and run a few miles or work up a sweat on a twenty-mile bike ride. The majority of studies agree it is not the type of exercise that matters as much as doing a form of activity or movement. Walking thirty minutes a day, most days a week, at moderate intensity, provides health benefits. Add in two days a week of strength training for even more benefits. As an alternative, mind-body therapies such as yoga and meditation have also been associated with decreased inflammation levels.[36]

If you're curious about your inflammation level, there is a simple blood test that can give you an idea. High sensitivity CRP (C-reactive protein) is a biomarker for inflammation levels in the body. The higher the CRP level, the higher the inflammation level. CRP level has been correlated with the risk of heart disease, with greater risk at levels greater than 3mg/L.[37]

---

[36] Julienne E. Bower and Michael R. Irwin, "Mind–body Therapies and Control of Inflammatory Biology: A Descriptive Review," Brain Behavior and Immunity 51 (January 2016): 1–11.

[37] Paul M. Ridker, "A Test in Context: High-Sensitivity C-Reactive Protein," Journal of the American College of Cardiology 67, no. 6 (2016): 712-723.

BOTTOM LINE

Stress unleashes trouble in the form of bad inflammation. Chronic inflammation and its troublemakers are one way that stress leads to disease. Troublemakers sensitize the nerves, leading to sensitization syndromes. Troublemakers also increase the risk of heart disease, stroke, and diabetes. Managing stress, a healthy diet, and regular exercise keep the troublemakers away.

CHAPTER 26

Tying it all together

AT THE BEGINNING OF THIS book, I explained that I chose *Sunbreak* for the title because, at the time I was writing it, I lived in the Pacific Northwest. Catching a glimpse of the sun breaking through the clouds reminds me of the light that comes with awareness. A glimmer of hope. The path toward healing.

I slowly improved from my stress-related disorder, although I haven't returned to my baseline. I've applied the strategies and actions described in *Sunbreak*. I made life changes that were critical to my healing. I had to take a close look at what I could sustain long-term. Twelve- to sixteen-hour work days were no longer realistic. Thirty-six-hour shifts were definitely not conceivable.

It's not easy to make major changes. Especially, when the changes make you feel you are letting others down. Healthy change begins with awareness and detachment from your ego's expectations.

Awareness, reducing stress, and learning to set boundaries were key for me. I decided to leave academic medicine. At that time, it was too difficult to stay within reasonable work boundaries. My people-pleasing tendencies did not serve me well in an environment with so many hefty demands. I decided that I needed more than glimmers of sun, so I moved to Arizona. I bought a home with tall windows and only one room with blinds. I'm surrounded by light. I bask in the sun each day; it's my daily vitamin. And some days, I skip sunscreen.

Recovery, your way

I've shared the journeys of Melissa, Bryan, Jenna and other individuals, each one on their own unique life path. Their common thread was that each developed and recovered from a different stress-related disorder.

Melissa's stress-related disorder was chronic low back pain with sensitization. Her symptoms were the end manifestation of multiple issues: stress, nerve sensitization, and arthritis.

The keys to her recovery were awareness of sensitization—what it was and how it affected her body. She also incorporated exercise and medication therapy. Melissa ultimately stepped away from her make-up business. She focused on caring for her two young children and worked a part-time job that was far less stressful. She improved significantly, however, she continues with medication therapy to manage her symptoms.

Jenna's stress-related disorder appeared as right-sided numbness, the result of a functional neurologic disorder. The key to her recovery was awareness of how stress was affecting her body. She used that knowledge to reduce the stressors in her life. Jenna was able to make adjustments to both her work schedule and her mom schedule. Reducing stress levels resolved frequent episodes of right-sided numbness. Her symptoms do recur on occasion, when stress levels become unmanageable. But now, Jenna knows the signs and the corrections she needs to make.

Bryan's stress-related disorder came in the form of chronic, agonizing headaches. Like Melissa and Jenna, Bryan began by learning how years of unrelenting stress had taken its toll on his body. And, like the others, he had to come to terms with making life changes.

His recovery began by reducing work stress, in combination with medication therapy to treat the painful headaches. He was able to continue his current business by hiring additional employees. He still needs daily medication to keep his headaches from returning, but Bryan has found a way to manage his headaches by understanding how stress impacts him physically.

Despite different life paths and conditions, their journeys to healing all contained the same key elements of awareness of their stress-body connection and identification and reduction of triggers.

> **" LISTEN TO YOUR BODY.**
> **SOMETIMES IT WHISPERS.**
> **SOMETIMES IT SCREAMS. "**

CHAPTER 27

Find the right provider for you

NOW THAT YOU UNDERSTAND STRESS-RELATED disorders and sensitization syndromes, how do you choose a provider who will collaborate with you? Not all providers are trained in sensitization syndromes. Not all providers have experience treating them. Finding the right provider for your specific needs is all about finding the right fit for you. The smartest doctor may not be the best fit for these conditions if they have no empathy. These conditions aren't that complicated, but you need someone who understands your struggle and that it's not just in your head. Well, it IS partially in your head, but only because your brain is in your head and that is where pain signals are processed!

Find a provider for your sensitization syndrome

Have you been wondering throughout this book how you can find a healthcare provider to help you with your sensitization syndrome? If you're suffering with a CSS—such as chronic headaches, back pain, or digestive issues—you need a professional who deals with ALL the aspects. Here are the key points the right provider should address:

- ☐ Considers the whole body. These are system-wide disorders. The right provider has you fill out a pain map—a visual of where all the pain is— that shows they are considering the whole picture and not being too narrowly focused.

- ☐ Asks about your non-pain symptoms (e.g., fatigue, brain fog, sleep issues).

- ☐ Evaluates your mental health, including a history of abuse or trauma.

☐ Actually examines you.

☐ Discusses the impact of stress, sleep, and exercise on your symptoms.

☐ Tailors a treatment to you, not according to a one-size-fits-all algorithm.

☐ Focuses on getting you back to the activities you enjoy and not just getting the pain score to zero.

☐ Asks about your functionality, like work and hobbies; these are key metrics for improvement from sensitization disorders.

☐ Promotes realistic expectations. Healing is a process that takes time.

☐ Maintains a network of associated providers to allow for complementary treatments, such as psychologists, physical therapists, chiropractors, acupuncturists, and massage therapists.

☐ Understands the type of medications useful in treating sensitization, including nerve pain agents.

Are we right for each other?

Knowledge and experience with CSS are essential in a healthcare provider treating a CSS. That's a great start, but you should also expect your doctor to possess certain character traits.

Here is a checklist of characteristics to look for when choosing your healthcare provider:

Empathy. Someone who is present and paying attention, a person who genuinely cares about your struggle. Look for a professional who truly listens and is not just waiting for their turn to talk, typing notes while you're talking but without ever looking at you. Find someone who does not interrupt you after five seconds. Someone who makes eye contact, who sees you.

Honest. You need someone who is not afraid to be truthful with you, who can handle an uncomfortable conversation. If you tell them all your symptoms and they just stare at you and change the subject or don't acknowledge your symptoms, that is a bad sign. If they are unsure, they should say so. If it's a delicate topic, the right provider is able to talk to you about it. I saw this commonly, providers afraid of offending patients so they don't tell them what is going on.

Communicative. Look for a provider who takes the time to explain what is going on with you and does not merely dictate what you should do. Your care should feel collaborative, based on your goals and values. Knowledge is power when understanding your health and how to heal. The right provider welcomes your questions and recognizes that you're committed to your health.

Consistent. New day, new doc clinics. Avoid clinics that schedule you with a different provider each time; you need to build rapport and a relationship with the person you're trusting with your care. You get better care from someone who knows your story, patterns, and nuances. When your provider leaves a practice or retires, do you just dread trying to find a new one? It's hard to find someone who understands your story and meets your needs, yet that's critical.

Open-minded. You owe it to yourself to find someone who isn't too righteous about Western medicine; complementary therapies have a role in helping various medical conditions. You can be both evidence-based and open-minded. Western medicine doesn't know it all! Completing randomized controlled trials on everything is not realistic, especially if the intervention isn't profitable for someone. Certain medical conditions are heavily studied while others are not. Regardless, you need treatment. Oftentimes, the science reasonably applies to multiple situations, especially for therapies used to manage symptoms.

Red flags = Move on

I've seen and worked with many healthcare providers. The experience has allowed me to see behavior patterns—specifically, those you should avoid. Here are some of those personalities and why you need to turn and run away from them.

Dr. Proceduralist keeps referring you to repeat procedures that didn't work the first few times. Remember Einstein's definition of insanity: "Insanity is doing the same thing over and over and expecting different results."

Dr. Inflexible is a provider who is too rigid or "black or white". Clinical medicine is shades of gray. Not everything can be studied and supported by randomized controlled trials; even fewer things can be studied accurately. If an action makes sense from a scientific standpoint and is low-risk, it is worth the provider being open and considering it.

Dr. Invalidator tells you that your experience isn't real or couldn't be, invalidating the reality you are living. A provider can't understand your struggle if they don't believe you. Without clear understanding and acceptance, they aren't going to provide the care you need.

Dr. Gaslighter talks down to you. They explain things with a condescending tone like you barely made it past kindergarten. They are attempting to make you feel ignorant, to doubt yourself, and do as they say without question. You go to a provider for advice, not manipulation and disrespect.

Dr. Narcissus acts like the visit is about their brilliance, not you. They expect you to be impressed just by having the opportunity to meet with them. They don't allow you to question their actions or decisions. The medical profession is teeming with narcissism. Dr. Narcissus is a cousin of Dr. Gaslighter.

Dr. Algorithm can't think beyond the guidelines. Patient care is not that simple. Guidelines are guidelines and not rules for a reason; they don't apply to everyone. If a provider can't see you are unique—not shove you into a computer-generated formula—they may be too rigid.

Dr. Brushoff ignores your symptoms. Your issue is not significant or not worth their time. If you don't have cancer or an infection, they don't care, it's below them. Do you want to waste your own time on a person like this?

Everyone's Miserable Medical Center is easily spotted. During your clinic visit, the receptionist, the medical assistant, and the nurse are rude, disinterested, and disrespectful. If everyone looks miserable in the office, they are. The clinic is toxic; don't catch the infection.

BOTTOM LINE

Listen to your intuition. You know when someone gets you and your struggle. And remember, second opinions are invaluable. There is surprising variation in treatment approaches among providers. If you feel uneasy, talk to another provider.

The reality is that not every clinician is a good fit for every person. Not every clinician is well-trained in your medical condition. And, not all providers are good clinicians; it's a spectrum from barely adequate to exceptional. Find the best fit so you get the quality of care that you need and deserve.

TOOL SUMMARY

Throughout *Sunbreak*, I have shared the tools I personally found helpful in healing from a stress-related disorder—my own and those of my patients. Tools that help build awareness and strengthen the mind-body connection to reduce symptoms. Here's a summary for easy reference.

Journaling:

- ☐ Awareness Journal—Pay attention to the signs and build your mind-body connection

- ☐ Thought Journal—Get your thoughts out of your head and process them at a deeper level

- ☐ Gratitude Journal—Tune your subconscious to the positive

Central Sensitization Inventory (CSI)— Improving awareness of nerve sensitization symptoms

Perceived Stress Scale—Understand your actual stress level

Stress Management Strategies:

- ☐ Social support from supportive people

- ☐ Regular exercise that you like on your schedule

- ☐ Expressive outlets and hobbies, scheduled into the week

- ☐ Sleep

- ☐ Mindfulness practice

Mental Health Symptoms and Awareness

- ☐ PHQ-9

- ☐ PHQ-15

- ☐ GAD-7

- ☐ Diaphragmatic breathing

ACKNOWLEDGEMENTS

To my better half, Regan Berschauer, thank you for supporting me during my best years, and supporting me even more during my worst.

Sue Publicover, I hired an editor, but I found a collaborative, dedicated, and brilliant writer, coach, and friend.

Sue, Voula Popovich, and Melissa Johnson thank you for balancing out Dr. Johnson's technical, dry science writing with Dr. Shana's person-focused explanations and tips.

Thank you to the beta readers and proofreaders for your honest feedback and perspectives that shaped *Sunbreak*: Celina Bronson, Susan Lyman, Lisa Moore, Lori Movsesian, Janis Urbanek, and Annette Wetherby.

To the design team, thank you Sarah Haynes and Shari Morton for bringing *Sunbreak* to life.

Thank you Debra Van Tuinen for your graciousness in providing the cover art for *Sunbreak*.

GLOSSARY

Acupuncture. An Eastern medical therapy that is delivered by tiny needles inserted into specific points in the body to bring balance to the nervous system; acupuncture may be used alone or in combination with medical therapy for a variety of sensitization syndromes.

Acute. A sudden onset, as in pain.

All-or-nothing thinking. A type of cognitive distortion in which an individual perceives themselves and the world around them in extremes, as good or bad, with no in-between.

Amygdala. A small, almond-shaped area in the brain that processes fearful and threatening stimuli; the amygdala also regulates anxiety, aggression, and fear conditioning.

Anhedonia. A reduced or complete inability to enjoy activities; a lack of interest or indifference to activities once enjoyed.

Anticonvulsants. Medications used for the prevention and treatment of seizures; also used for conditions unrelated to seizures, particularly nerve pain.

Anxiety disorder (generalized anxiety disorder). A mental health condition characterized by excessive, uncontrollable and frequent worry; worrisome thoughts are difficult to control and interfere with day-to-day activities.

Autonomic nervous system. The part of the nervous system that controls automatic functions of the body, such as heart rate and breathing; consists of the sympathetic nervous system (fight-or-flight response) and the parasympathetic nervous system (rest and digest response).

Awareness Journal. A book for writing thoughts in order to connect stress and other triggers with physical symptoms; the awareness journaling process helps build the mind-body connection.

Beta blocker. A medication prescribed to treat various conditions—including heart conditions and headaches—providing relief by reducing the effects of adrenaline.

Brain fog. A non-medical term used to describe difficulty concentrating and thinking clearly.

Cannabinoids. A group of substances found in the cannabis plant; two well-known cannabinoids are tetrahydrocannabinol (THC) and cannabidiol (CBD).

Central sensitization inventory. A clinical assessment tool used to measure the symptoms associated with central sensitization.

Central sensitization syndromes (CSS). A group of medical conditions that share the common abnormality of nerve sensitization; sensitization causes the nerves to be over-reactive and contributes to a variety of chronic pain disorders, such as headaches, back pain, and digestive issues.

Chronic. Recurring or persisting for an extended period.

Chronic low-grade inflammation. Acute inflammation occurs after an injury or infection and helps the body to heal; with chronic inflammation, immune cells stay active in the absence of injury which is harmful to the body.

Cognitive behavioral therapy (CBT). A form of psychotherapy that works on promoting healthy thought patterns and reducing cognitive distortions (biased thought patterns).

Cognitive distortion. Thinking patterns that are inaccurate and often negatively biased.

Conversion disorder. Neurologic symptoms, such as numbness or weakness, that present without a neurologic explanation—e.g., no tumor or stroke causing the symptoms. Frequently, conversion is precipitated by an acute stressor, trauma, or adverse life event. The physical symptoms are not consciously controlled by the person. Also referred to as functional neurologic disorder.

Detachment. To separate or distance from something.

Diaphragmatic breathing. A form of slow, deep breathing that turns off the stress response, calming the nervous system.

Disordered pain processing. Pain signals that are not interpreted normally by the brain, spinal cord, and nerves; pain signals perceived in the brain are not accurate.

Dysfunction. Abnormality in function.

Emotional reasoning. A cognitive distortion in which a person draws conclusions based on their feelings and emotions; for example, feeling like a failure and then concluding to be a failure, rather than recognizing it as a feeling. See cognitive distortion.

Emotional regulation. The ability to exert control over one's own emotional state; to be aware of emotions and respond to them in a healthy way.

Enteric nervous system. A network of nerves in the gastrointestinal tract that control its functions.

Equanimity. A state of calmness and composure, maintained even in difficult situations.

Fibromyalgia. A central sensitization syndrome characterized by widespread body pain.

Fight-or-flight response. A term for the activation of the body's stress response due to a perceived threat.

Functional MRI. Functional magnetic resonance imaging; a test that shows what areas of the brain are active during certain tasks, such as picking up objects or feeling pain.

Functional neurologic disorder (FND). Neurologic symptoms, such as numbness or weakness, without a neurologic explanation—e.g., no tumor or stroke causing the symptoms. Frequently, FND is precipitated by an acute stressor, trauma, or adverse life event. The physical symptoms are not consciously controlled by the person. Also referred to as conversion disorder.

Gut. The digestive tract, including the stomach and intestines.

Interstitial cystitis. A central sensitization syndrome characterized by chronic bladder pain.

Irritable bowel syndrome. A central sensitization syndrome affecting the digestive tract with chronic abdominal pain, cramping, constipation, and/or diarrhea.

Ketamine. A medication used as an anesthetic agent and also illicitly as a hallucinogen; currently under study for use in depression and central sensitization pain.

Limbic system. The emotional center of the brain.

Magnification and minimization. A type of cognitive distortion in which a person magnifies the negative and minimizes the positive aspects of a situation. See cognitive distortion.

Mental filtering. A cognitive distortion in which the individual dwells on the negative details of a situation and ignores or discounts the positive. See cognitive distortion.

Meta-awareness. The ability to detach from your immediate experience and be an objective observer of the experience.

Metabolic syndrome. A group of conditions that together raise the risk for cardiovascular disease—including obesity, high blood pressure, high blood sugar, and cholesterol abnormalities.

Mindfulness. The state of being aware of feelings, thoughts, and actions in the present moment.

Mixed pain state. A condition in which multiple sources of pain develop; for example, pain arising from an injured area, like the back, and pain from disordered sensory processing.

Myofascial pain syndrome. A central sensitization syndrome with chronic muscle pain and tenderness in a region of the body, such as the upper back.

Negative rumination. Repetitive negative thinking.

Nerve sensitization. Health condition that arises from abnormalities in the way that pain signals are processed and perceived in the nervous system; nerves are more sensitive and reactive to stimuli, which increases the pain signal perceived.

Nerve stimulator. A type of medical device used to treat nerve pain.

Neurocircuitry. The arrangement of neurons and their connections in the nervous system.

Neurodivergent. Neurodivergence considers that people experience and interact with the world around them in a variety of ways with differences in thinking, learning, and behavior; often used in the context of autism spectrum disorder as well as other neurological differences such as ADHD or learning disabilities.

Neuroinflammation. Inflammation in the nervous system.

Neurologic disorder. A medical condition arising from dysfunction in the nervous system.

Neuropathic agents. Medications used to treat sensitization and nerve pain.

Neuropathic pain. Pain that arises from direct damage to the nerves.

Nociceptive pain. Pain caused by inflammation and tissue damage.

Nociplastic pain. Pain that comes from abnormal pain processing in the nervous system.

Overgeneralization. A cognitive distortion in which a person makes a broad conclusion about themself based on a single event; for example, failure at one task is generalized to failure at all tasks. See cognitive distortion.

Pain hypersensitivity. Increased sensitivity to sensory inputs, such as touch, pressure, and movement.

Patient health questionnaire 9 (PHQ-9). A clinical assessment tool used to measure depression symptoms.

Perceived Stress Scale. A clinical assessment tool that measures an individual's perceived level of stress.

Placebo effect. A positive treatment effect resulting from a person's anticipation that the treatment will work.

Prefrontal cortex (PFC). The area of the brain that helps to regulate thoughts, actions, and emotions, as well as assisting with insight, reasoning, and decision-making.

Propranolol. A type of beta blocker. See beta blocker.

Psychedelics. A type of substance that alters a person's perception of reality; recently, under study for use in treating mental health conditions and pain.

Randomized controlled trial. A study design that randomly assigns participants into a treatment group or a control group. The use of randomization reduces bias and is the best way to examine cause and effect relationships between a treatment and outcome.

SNRI (serotonin and norepinephrine reuptake inhibitors). A class of medications that increase the amount of serotonin and norepinephrine in the brain—messengers that help with mood and pain.

Somatization. Physical symptoms that are part of the expression of a mental health condition.

Stress hormone. A hormone, such as adrenaline or cortisol, that is released in response to stress. See fight-or-flight response.

Stress response. The physiological changes that occur in the body as the result of a perceived threat; the response developed to improve survival from an immediate physical threat. During the stress response, stress hormones are released that increase heart rate and breathing while decreasing digestion and repair. See fight-or-flight response.

Stress-related disorder. A medical condition that is triggered or worsened by high levels of stress.

System-wide symptoms. Symptoms that impact the entire body.

Temporomandibular joint disorder. A sensitization syndrome characterized by pain and tenderness in the jaw joint.

Thalamus. A part of the brain responsible for relaying pain information, among other functions.

Tricyclics. A medication class originally used to treat depression and found to be useful in treating neuropathic and sensitization pain. See neuropathic agent.

INDEX

ABOUT THE AUTHOR

Dr. Shana Johnson is a board-certified physician in physical medicine and re-habilitation. Over the past twenty years, she has cared for people with conditions affecting the brain, spine, and nerves. Multiple sclerosis was a particular focus of hers and she spent time as the co-director of a multiple sclerosis clinic. She also cared for people with brain injuries, spinal cord injuries, and strokes. And pain of all different types–back pain, headaches, and whole-body pain.

Over the years, Dr. Shana noticed a different patient group, a staggering number of people who developed medical conditions while under unrelenting stress—disorders such as chronic headaches, back pain, and digestive issues. People came to Dr. Shana for help, after enduring years of ineffective procedures and medication trials. The connection to stress and its role in treatment was rarely acknowledged or addressed, so people just lived with their conditions.

Dr. Shana, who suffered the same problem, wrote *Sunbreak: Healing the pain no one can explain* to shine a light on stress-related disorders and provide a resource for those struggling with them.

Dr. Shana lives in Arizona with her husband and son.